T0219893

RESEARCH DURING MEDICAL RESIDENCY

RESEARCH DURING MEDICAL RESIDENCY

A How-To Guide for Residents
and Faculty Mentors

Lynne M. Bianchi Ph.D.
Director of Medical Research Operations
Medical Research Center
University of Pittsburgh Medical Center (UPMC)
Hamot and Gannon University

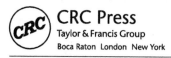

CRC Press
Taylor & Francis Group
Boca Raton London New York

CRC Press is an imprint of the
Taylor & Francis Group, an **informa** business

First edition published 2022
by CRC Press
6000 Broken Sound Parkway NW, Suite 300, Boca Raton, FL 33487-2742

and by CRC Press
4 Park Square, Milton Park, Abingdon, Oxon, OX14 4RN
CRC Press is an imprint of Taylor & Francis Group, LLC

Library of Congress Cataloging-in-Publication Data

Names: Bianchi, Lynne M. (Professor of neuroscience), editor.
Title: Research during medical residency : a how-to guide for residents and faculty mentors / edited by Lynne M. Bianchi.
Description: First edition. | Boca Raton : CRC Press, 2022. | Includes bibliographical references and index. | Summary: "This book is a guide for medical residents and faculty in the fundamentals of clinical research, publication practices, and conference skills. It offers advice on how to incorporate scholarly activities into training routines, so the process becomes more manageable and less overwhelming. Suggestions for pursuing other scholarly activities, outside of clinical research, are also offered. Participation in research and other scholarly activities is a requirement for graduation from medical residency programs in the United States and many other countries. Faculty physicians who train residents are also required to produce annual scholarly work. Adding scholarship onto an already long list of requirements often feels a bit daunting to medical residents and the faculty who teach them. Fortunately, there are many forms of scholarly activity including basic and clinical research, quality improvement projects, and educational assessments so everyone can find interesting and feasible projects to complete. This valuable reference provides users a reliable source to turn to whenever they have questions on how to develop, conduct, publish, or present a research project. Written with the perspective of busy faculty and residents in mind, the content balances the need for enough detail to be instructive with the need for quick access to key points"-- Provided by publisher.
Identifiers: LCCN 2021051999 (print) | LCCN 2021052000 (ebook) | ISBN 9780367648305 (paperback) | ISBN 9780367648336 (hardback) | ISBN 9781003126478 (ebook)
Subjects: MESH: Biomedical Research--methods | Medical Writing | Internship and Residency | Speech | Mentors
Classification: LCC R852 (print) | LCC R852 (ebook) | NLM W 20.5 | DDC 610.72/4--dc23/eng/20211130
LC record available at https://lccn.loc.gov/2021051999
LC ebook record available at https://lccn.loc.gov/2021052000]

ISBN: 9780367648336 (hbk)
ISBN: 9780367648305 (pbk)
ISBN: 9781003126478 (ebk)

DOI: 10.1201/9781003126478

Typeset in Times
by Deanta Global Publishing Services, Chennai, India

To our mentors, mentees, and families, with
appreciation for all they have taught us.

Contents

Preface

The idea for this book came during my second year as Director of Medical Research at a community-based hospital. Part of residency training includes participation in scholarly activities such as research, quality improvement projects, and educational innovations. However, residents and their faculty mentors often find it difficult to balance clinical practice and scholarship. In discussions with the residency program directors and senior residents, common needs were identified and the concept of a "handy little book" covering essential material in a practical way emerged.

The goal of this book is to make every step of the scholarly process, from idea development to data dissemination, more manageable and less confusing. The book offers unique perspectives, as co-authors include those with extensive scholarly experience and those with less experience, an approach used to ensure information important for new investigators was identified and highlighted in each chapter.

We hope this book serves as a valuable resource and allows residents and faculty to discover the many ways to simplify scholarly activity, incorporate projects into daily practice, and more readily balance the demands of clinical and scholarly work.

Lynne M. Bianchi

Acknowledgments

The authors thank the residents and faculty at the University of Pittsburgh Medical Center (UPMC), Hamot for their input on chapter topics. Special thanks to Patricia Ladds, Samantha Cascone, Annmarie Kutz, Karen Martin, and Michalle Schodt of the Medical Education Department for their enthusiastic support throughout this project. Thanks to Diann Cooper for her helpful comments on early chapter drafts. The author thanks Chuck Crumly for taking interest in the project and sharing the idea with Miranda Bromage. It has been a pleasure to work with Miranda throughout the process. Many thanks to Miranda, Samantha Cook, Linda Leggio, and Jayanthi Chander for all of their help and guidance in preparing the final manuscript.

Contributors

Joyce Babyak, Ph.D.
Religion Department
Oberlin College
Oberlin, OH

Sean Carroll, D.O.
Department of Otolaryngology—Head
and Neck Surgery
University of Pittsburgh Medical Center,
Hamot
Erie, PA

Diann C. Cooper, Ph.D., M.S.N., R.N., B.C.
Villa Maria School of Nursing
Gannon University
Erie, PA

Calhoun D. Cunningham III, M.D.
Department of Head and Neck Surgery &
Communication Sciences
Duke University School of Medicine
Raleigh, NC

James DeLullo, M.D.
Department of Orthopaedic Surgery
Residency Program Director
University of Pittsburgh Medical Center,
Hamot
Erie, PA

Jeffrey Esper, D.O.
Neurology Department
University of Pittsburgh Medical Center,
Hamot
Erie, PA

Dominik Greda, M.D.
Premier ENT Associates
Miami Valley Hospital
South Centerville, OH

Randy Jeffrey, M.D., Ph.D.
Department of Cardiology
University of Pittsburgh Medical Center,
Hamot
Erie, PA

Kristin Juhasz, D.O.
Department of Emergency Medicine
University of Pittsburgh Medical Center,
Hamot
Erie, PA

Ajaipal S. Kang, M.D.
Department of Plastic and Reconstructive
Surgery
University of Pittsburgh Medical Center,
Hamot
Erie, PA

Annmarie Kutz, M.S.
Otolaryngology—Head and Neck
Surgery
Department of Medical Education
University of Pittsburgh Medical Center,
Hamot
Erie, PA

John D. Lubahn, M.D.
Department of Orthopaedic
Surgery
University of Pittsburgh Medical Center,
Hamot
Erie, PA

Robert Maholic, D.O.
Interventional Cardiology
University of Pittsburgh Medical Center,
Hamot
Erie, PA

Trevor Phinney, D.O.
Neurology Department
University of Pittsburgh Medical Center,
   Hamot
Erie, PA

Justin Puller, M.D.
Department of Emergency Medicine
University of Pittsburgh Medical Center,
   Hamot
Erie, PA

Luke J. Rosielle, Ph.D.
Department of Psychology and Counselling
Gannon University
Erie, PA

Alice Wang, M.D.
Premier Weight Loss Solutions
Premier Health
Dayton, OH

Introduction: Developing Ways to Incorporate Scholarly Activity into Clinical Training and Practice

Lynne M. Bianchi, Ph.D. and Justin Puller, M.D.

Tips for Success:

> Choose a form of scholarly activity that fits your personality, interests, and resources.
> Develop projects that are attractive to you and beneficial to your field.
> Design studies that can be completed given your available resources.
> Spend time reading the literature.

Warnings:

> It takes a bit of effort to develop an idea into a worthwhile project.
> Ideas are revised multiple times before implementing a project.

Key Concept: Planning may feel like wasted time but planning always saves time and prevents frustration.

Life during medical residency includes a variety of anticipated and unanticipated activities and experiences. There is a lot to learn and master in a short period of time. Most new residents expect long hours, difficult cases, challenging supervisors, and a lack of sleep. Many know they will attend and give lectures and spend time preparing for exams. Some, however, are surprised to discover they also must engage in research. If one matches into a residency program at a large medical university known for cutting-edge research, it is likely that the person wanted to include research training as part of the residency experience. For those who select residencies in community-based hospitals, rural settings, or programs not affiliated with a medical school, the requirement to engage in research may come as a bit of a surprise, a sense of dread, or perhaps the thought, "they won't really make me do that, will they?" Yet, **participation in research and other scholarly activities is a requirement for graduation from residency programs** in the United States and many other countries. **Faculty physicians** who train residents are also required to produce annual scholarly work.

DOI: 10.1201/9781003126478-1

Adding scholarship onto an already long list of requirements often feels a bit overwhelming to residents and the faculty who teach them. Fortunately, there are **many forms of scholarly activity**, including **basic and clinical research**, **quality improvement** projects, and **educational assessments**, so everyone can find something interesting to do (**Box 1.1**).

We designed this book to guide residents and faculty in the fundamentals of clinical research, publication practices, and conference skills. We offer advice on how to incorporate scholarly activities into your weekly routine, so the process becomes more manageable and less onerous. Suggestions for pursuing other scholarly activities, outside of clinical research, are also offered.

Remember: To be a successful scholar, one does not have to work at a laboratory bench or develop a novel clinical therapy. One does not need to publish in a top medical journal or speak at the most prestigious subspecialty conference. **One simply needs to identify interesting questions, implement appropriate ways to answer them, and share their outcomes through presentations or publications**.

Note: Throughout this book, discussions of **"projects"** and **"studies" refer to all forms of scholarship**, not just clinical research studies. Similarly, the terms "investigator" and "researcher" refer to those involved in any scholarly project.

Tip: Scholarly activity supports the culture of inquiry needed to advance medical knowledge and improve patient care.

Hint: If you consider scholarly work meaningless to your clinical practice, periodically remind yourself of the inherent connection between scholarly activity and patient care.

Box 1.1   The Many Forms of Scholarly Activities: Choose What Works for You and Plan Accordingly

In addition to clinical research, scholarly activities include **quality improvement** (QI) or **quality assurance** (QA) projects, and **education assessments** (see References and Resources).

In the United States, the Accreditation Council for Graduate Medical Education (ACGME) requires annual scholarly activity reports from residents and their faculty mentors (Tables 1.1 and 1.2). Programs in other countries have their own guidelines and requirements.

Due to the nature of scholarship, no individual produces work in every category each year. For residents and faculty reporting to the ACGME, most list accomplishments in different categories annually. For example, a **resident** may participate in teaching in year one, start working on a research project in year two, and present a poster in year three. A **faculty** member might receive a grant,

Table 1.1 ACGME Resident Scholarly Activities

1. Publications with PMID	4. Chapters in textbooks
2. Other publications	5. Participated in research (Yes/No)
3. Conference presentations	6. Teaching presentations (Yes/No)

All residents and fellows must participate in scholarly activity prior to graduation. Six categories of scholarly activity are recorded for each resident or fellow annually. The identification number(s) for publications cited in PubMed (the PMID) are listed, and the total number of other publications and the number of presentations at regional, national, or international conferences are reported. Whether the resident participated in research or teaching is also noted.

Table 1.2 ACGME Faculty Scholarly Activities

1. Publications with PMID	6. Chapters or textbooks
2. Peer-reviewed publications without a PMID	7. Grants with leadership role (e.g., Principal Investigator (PI), Co-PI, site director) Yes/No
3. Non peer-reviewed publications, item writing (e.g., board exam questions)	8. Leadership role in international, national, state, regional medical organizations; reviewer or editorial board of peer-reviewed journal Yes/No
4. Conference presentations	9. Coordinator of seminars, conference series, or courses for medical students, residents, fellows, or other health
5. Other presentations (e.g., Grand Rounds, invited lectures)	professionals outside of program didactics/conferences Yes/No

For faculty, the annual report to the ACGME includes a chart with nine categories. All PMIDs are listed in the first category. The number of other publications and presentations are then listed under the appropriate categories (categories 2–6). Faculty also indicate whether they held grant leadership, committee leadership, or peer-review roles, or coordinated formal conferences or courses outside of their residency program. Details of what activities to include under each category are listed in ACGME Common Program Requirements (see References and Resources).

PMID (PubMed Identification number): the number assigned to articles listed in the PubMed database (see Chapter 2).

present posters on that work for two years, then publish a paper. Another may be involved in peer review each year, co-author a poster with residents annually, and publish a new book chapter every few years. A third might give Grand Round lectures and coordinate a course every year, and periodically present or publish on projects related to assessment of learning outcomes. Some may prefer to focus on QI projects and regularly present findings at regional meetings. Thus, **there are many ways to meet the requirements simply by pursuing areas of interest**.

It is always helpful to **track your expected accomplishments to ensure you meet annual program and institutional requirements**.

Depending on the specialty and institutional requirements, residents or fellows may be expected to present at a conference, prepare a manuscript for publication, or write a literature review.

Note: Residents and faculty should **work with the program director and program coordinator** to identify acceptable forms of scholarly activity and **establish timelines for completion.**

Tip: Check that you will have **at least one form of scholarly activity completed by the eighth month of each academic year.** If you discover you do not have any scholarly activities for that year, you will have four months to accomplish something relevant.

Hint: You are unlikely to complete a new scholarly activity in the final weeks of the academic year. Plan accordingly.

1.1 TURN YOUR INTERESTS INTO SCHOLARLY WORK

The first step to developing sustainable scholarly work is to choose projects that readily integrate into your weekly routine. New investigators may overlook this critical concept and fret unnecessarily over the prospect of creating a new project unrelated to anything else they do. One of the most important lessons in this book is that **successful scholarly activity arises as a natural extension of your daily work and interests.** For example, if a program director is revising curricular content, projects that assess teaching methods or learning outcomes can be initiated. If residents devote several hours to a community service initiative, research or educational projects tied to that initiative can be developed. **There is no need to invent extra work unrelated to your current interests and efforts.**

CONSIDER THE QUESTIONS YOU ASK AND THE INTERESTS YOU HAVE

Every week, you wonder about many different things. Simply being an engaged clinician leads you to ask questions. Think about some of your recent questions or observations. Do you question whether a newer, expensive medication benefits patients more than the older, inexpensive version? Do you believe second-year residents need additional training in aspects of hospital procedure? Have you wondered if transportation barriers influence which patients receive follow-up care? Do you suspect residents who regularly visit the art museum are better at reading patient body language? Such **everyday questions can often form the foundation of a scholarly project.**

Note, however, that even if you ask several important questions each day, if you are not motivated to discover the answers, then you are unlikely to complete any projects designed to answer them. That may seem obvious, but many investigators start with questions they think they *should* answer, then quickly lose interest. With so much going on each day, uninteresting projects are easy to set aside. **Focus your efforts on projects that leave you truly curious about the outcome.**

If you are unsure where or how to begin, **start with broader interests**, such as a specific disease or condition, a particular patient age-group, or a clinical procedure. Consider the approaches used in descriptive clinical studies, experimental controlled trials, basic science experiments, community-based initiatives, and hospital quality improvement projects. **Identify approaches that appeal to you**. Some investigators prefer basic science questions and enjoy working quietly in a lab tinkering with reagents and gadgets. Others loathe the thought of working in a lab, alone or otherwise, and prefer clinical observational studies or quality improvement projects.

Everyone has **preferred ways of thinking and working**. As you consider different projects, remember to **focus on the questions and approaches that fit your interests, personality, and work style**.

When you talk to experienced, successful researchers, it is easy to detect their enthusiasm. Without passion for their work, they could not sustain their efforts. One could not devote 20 years to studying the molecular signaling pathways governing development of the embryonic forebrain if one did not enjoy thinking about molecular signaling pathways governing development of the embryonic forebrain. To many, such work would seem boring at best, but to those who study the topic, it is energizing. Perhaps you do not find the molecular signaling pathways of anything interesting, but you are interested in many topics. Start with some of those as you consider projects to pursue.

Keep in mind that **passion develops over time**. As you incorporate scholarly activities into your career, your interests evolve. However, do not be surprised or discouraged if you do not find a passion the first few times you engage in scholarly work. Start with an area that appeals to you and let your interests develop from there.

Also note that your interests will likely shift over time. Some interests shift quickly. A topic that appears interesting may seem less intriguing once the literature is read. Alternatively, a topic that sounds dreadfully boring may become exciting once you start thinking about how to design a study to find missing information.

Other interests change over longer periods. You may discover that questions that motivated you during an early-career stage are less intriguing at subsequent stages, or that the approaches you preferred as a resident do not work well when you are a senior clinician. Fortunately, scholarly work can always be adapted to fit your evolving interests, preferred approaches, and work schedule.

Tip: Start with a topic of some interest and learn how to do research. The more you do, the easier it becomes to identify projects that hold your interest. It also becomes easier to recognize projects that do *not* fit your interests, schedule, resources, or ways of thinking.

Hint: Keep a dedicated notebook. Add ideas that come to mind, even ones you may never pursue. List methods to consider, materials you would need, and questions to ask others. Add information about relevant articles, including strengths and weaknesses and areas that remain to be investigated.

MERGE INTERESTS WITH LOCAL NEEDS AND AVAILABLE RESOURCES
The projects you ultimately pursue will be influenced by (1) the **needs** of your **institution** and the surrounding **community** and (2) the **resources available**. Asking how your interests blend with local needs and available resources will help you refine your questions into **meaningful and manageable projects**.

Because **scholarly activity is the foundation for improving patient care**, it makes sense to focus efforts on local needs. Some new investigators try to mimic studies at other institutions without considering whether such studies fit their own institution or community populations. Some feel a study focused on local needs will not be of interest to the wider medical community. However, your findings may be relevant to those who work with similar populations or your approach might be adapted to suit other groups. Thus, developing projects that align with local needs is a practical and valuable form of scholarship. **The best way to develop projects that benefit your institution and surrounding community is to reflect on the questions that arise while engaged in patient care.**

As you consider various interests, identify which projects are most likely to succeed given your current or future resources. **Resources** include **time**, **personnel**, **equipment**, **supplies**, and **financial support**. Consider your present situation and your likely situation over the next one to two years. Which projects could you start in the next six months? Which projects would take more than a year to initiate?

Questions to consider include:

a) **Time**:
 - How will I incorporate a research project into my weekly schedule?
 - Will my availability change during the next year?
 - Will I have protected time to devote to scholarly activities/research? If so, how much?
b) **Personnel**:
 - Who is available to assist me with the project?
 - Are there residents, medical students, or pre-medical students who could work on the project?
 - Are there technicians, clinical staff, or clerical staff to assist?
 - Will available personnel be able to complete tasks on their own or will some need supervision?

c) **Physical resources**:
- What space, equipment, and supplies are readily available?
- Could I access additional physical resources if necessary?

d) **Financial resources**:
- Will I be given funds to complete a project? If so, how much? How do I access those funds?
- Do I need to apply for grant funds to support the project? If so, where can I apply? When are proposals due?

It is important to **be realistic in your assessment of available resources**. The best ideas cannot be developed into successful projects if resources are lacking.

Tip: If any resources are lacking, discuss your ideas with others to see if there are alternative ways to acquire what you need. If not, consider ways to refine your project to fit your existing resources.

Hint: **Start small**, have success with "easy" projects and move on from there. This gives you time to master skills, present and publish good work, and build a reputation as a careful and thoughtful investigator.

1.2 WORK WITH OTHERS TO DEVELOP A PROJECT

Both new and experienced investigators find it beneficial to work with others, particularly when initiating projects in a new area. Working with others ranges from participating in someone else's ongoing research to trouble-shooting ideas with colleagues. You will likely interact with other investigators in various ways at different times in your career.

JOIN AN EXISTING RESEARCH GROUP

One way to quickly get involved in research is to join a group that has an active research program. The lead investigator may have a list of projects to initiate, an ongoing study that requires final data collection, or a new idea to pursue. Although you may be restricted to projects unrelated to your primary interests, the experience will help you **develop skills needed for future projects**.

FOSTER COLLABORATIONS

Another way for new investigators to get started quickly is to collaborate with another investigator, preferably someone with more research experience. You might work with colleagues in your department, another department, or another institution. **Collaborations** require both parties to contribute ideas and resources to the project; **each investigator brings something the other lacks**. Examples of collaborations include: a resident with a month of research time helping a collaborator to process and analyze tissue samples; a faculty member without access to enough study participants at their hospital collaborating with colleagues at another hospital serving the target population; a faculty member interested in using cell culture assays working with a scientist at a local university.

Collaborations work well when all parties communicate regularly and follow through on their respective tasks. It is important to define roles at the beginning of a project as collaborations become challenging when individuals have different expectations about what each party will contribute. It is also important to work with those who are reliable and trustworthy. Because **all team members are accountable for the integrity of the data**, only collaborate with ethical individuals who will pay attention to all aspects of the project.

Discuss Ideas with Experienced Colleagues

Sharing your ideas with another investigator clarifies your plans and helps sort out potential weaknesses and complications. If no one at your institution is available, reach out to faculty at your former medical school, contact scientists at a local university, or request a mentor through a professional society.

Most experienced investigators are happy to share tips, give feedback on a project design, or read a draft of a grant proposal. No one is going to re-design your project or re-write your proposal, but most are willing to **help troubleshoot ideas and provide guidance when needed**.

Tip: Formal **mentorship programs for residents and junior faculty** are often sponsored by **professional societies**.

1.3 DEVELOP A PROJECT WITH ONE CLEAR AND SPECIFIC GOAL

Developing a good project begins by exploring broad ideas. Several tentative ideas are considered before the final project is defined (**Box 1.2**).

To develop a realistic and useful project, consider how your various ideas align with the **FINER criteria**. "FINER" stands for: Feasible, Interesting, Novel, Ethical, Relevant. Your project must be **feasible** given your resources, skills, and time. It should be **interesting**, not just to you, but to others in your field. It needs to be **novel**, filling a gap in knowledge. It may be a small gap, but there must be something unknown that would be interesting to figure out. The project must be **ethical** and abide by all regulations to protect participants. Your project must also be **relevant**. It helps to ask: "If my study finds what I expect it to find, what would that mean?" "Who would care about these results?" Some people refer to relevancy as the "So what?" question.

Note, there are projects that are feasible, interesting, novel, and ethical but irrelevant. Your project does not have to lead to a paradigm-shifting discovery, but it should add something useful to the medical community. You may leave new gaps, but you must add some relevant new knowledge.

It is important to stress that FINER criteria are not met in one afternoon of planning. It is equally important to note that **developing your project does not require several months of planning**. The time required to develop a project will depend on many factors, including how much *focused* time you dedicate to reading the literature and developing a project that meets FINER criteria. If you try to do this in fleeting moments between your other responsibilities, you will find yourself frustrated and convinced you do not have time for research.

Box 1.2   Finding a Single Focused Question

Imagine you are interested in the presumptive association between cognitive decline and age-related hearing loss. The literature suggests age-related hearing loss increases the chances of experiencing cognitive decline. You might decide to study whether hearing aid use decreases the risk of cognitive decline. However, you suspect that educational level is linked to hearing aid use and wonder if you should study the relationship between hearing aids, education, and cognitive decline. You also note that hearing aids are expensive and rarely covered by insurance which leads you to question if socioeconomic factors contribute to cognitive decline in older adults with hearing loss. You also wonder about the age of the hearing aids being used by those with and without cognitive decline. Is there something about the individuals who use the latest technology that lessens the chances of developing cognitive decline? You might question whether extended family members influence who uses hearing aids or who experiences cognitive decline.

Each of these questions has the potential to become a single, focused, research question. Existing data, your interests, and available resources will influence how you shape your questions into a feasible project. You may find that some of your ideas have already been explored in previous studies and thus you would rework your plans based on existing data. You may note that you could not adequately control for confounding variables, and so discard some plans. You might discover you do not have access to the population you need. Ultimately, you settle on a single, meaningful question that can be answered with your available resources.

Hint: Even when a study has multiple parts and several outcomes to consider, the project must be based on a single focused question.

1.4 IDENTIFY WEAKNESSES AND COMPLICATIONS BEFORE YOU BEGIN

Once you define your study question and methods, be sure to **discuss your plans with others before you begin**. Talk with colleagues early in the process to hone your idea, then discuss your revised plans to make sure you have not overlooked anything.

Ideally, you will discuss your project with those in the same field. However, that is not always possible, especially if you are in a smaller department or your idea is unrelated to other research at your institution. However, discussing your ideas with others is **beneficial, even if they are not experts in the topic area**. If your ideas make sense, others will be able to understand them easily; if others do not understand your proposed project, there is something wrong with your plans or how you present them.

Some colleagues will ask questions regarding background information; you should be able to answer those. If you cannot, note the areas you need to review. Other colleagues might ask about methods, control groups, or alternative ways to address your question. These types of questions may identify areas of weakness and help you refine your approach.

While it is **always nice to have colleagues say your ideas are great**, it is **not particularly helpful**. Be sure to discuss your project with those who will take the time to think through your idea, ask questions, identify weaknesses, and suggest alternatives.

Before you launch any study, **think about what it will take to complete the project successfully.** For example, if your study requires three years to complete, will there be research personnel available for the duration of the project? Is the study population readily available or will it take several years to recruit the required number of participants? Will you have the funds, personnel, and time to carry out the project for a longer period if necessary?

As noted above, there may be times when it is necessary to **revise** a study plan **to match available resources**. If your first plan cannot be completed with available resources, what is the next best option? Would reaching out to a collaborator with the necessary resources be advisable?

Remember: One should always design the best, most thorough study possible and aim to publish in the highest-quality journals. However, it is also helpful to note that **as a resident or new investigator, most projects will make smaller contributions to the field, and that is fine**. A small, well-designed, well-conducted study provides valuable research training and often generates preliminary data that justifies future research. What is most important is that the contribution, however small, be useful and accurate. Like most skills acquired during residency, research skills will grow over time and mostly flourish at later career stages.

Tip: **Consult with a statistician** to check that the study design and data collection plans are appropriate *before* you begin any study.

1.5 READ TO OPTIMIZE YOUR STUDY PLANS
New investigators may not appreciate that **reading is integral to the success of every project**. As you read the literature, you become an expert on your topic

and develop a fuller appreciation for the nuances of the field. This knowledge, in turn, helps you identify clear and specific goals that address important, missing information.

Through reading, your ideas and plans evolve. You might discover new approaches to better address your question, or you may stumble on a new area of focus. **Reading helps you refine your ideas into interesting and feasible studies**.

Note: **Good studies are not sudden flashes of inspiration that pop into one's head in a dream**. They come from understanding what is known, recognizing what is missing, and identifying ways to fill in that missing information. A dream-based inspiration may occur for some, but only because they read about the topic when awake.

Tip: As you read other studies, **note which study designs** and **variables are likely to provide the information you seek**.

Hint: See Chapter 4 for information on study designs and variables.

ACCEPT THAT READING REQUIRES DEDICATED TIME AND ATTENTION

To be successful in any scholarly activity, you must find time to read. **Set aside a specific period each week and stick to it**. The advice to set aside dedicated time for reading is one of those suggestions that most agree is a good idea, but few do. Yet, everyone who sets aside dedicated, focused time for reading quickly recognizes the benefits, and wonders why it was not done sooner. **You can find some time during the week to read**. You might use half an hour one morning or evening to identify articles and then set aside two hours on another day to read them. Perhaps you prefer a four-hour block once a week or maybe you process information better in smaller, more frequent periods, such as one hour each day. **The schedule that helps you to comprehend and retain information is the one to use**.

To read effectively, one must process what the authors present. There are big differences between skimming and active reading. Skimming through abstracts and articles is useful to get an overview of a topic and identify emerging areas of interest in a field. However, to fully understand a topic, improve a project idea, and develop appropriate methods, active, critical reading is required. **Critical reading involves** consideration of the data presented and the authors' interpretations. It involves **thinking about how the study design influenced the results** and **how the results fit into existing knowledge** (see Chapter 3).

Hint: A half-hour of reading each week will never be enough; although, with **practice**, the **time and effort required to digest a new article will decrease**.

Remember: Reading continues throughout all stages of a project. You **need different things from the literature at different times**. In the beginning, reading is primarily to gather background information and develop expertise. As you develop your study, you often go back to some papers to reconsider the methods or re-evaluate an author's interpretation. At the end of a study, you will review additional literature related to your findings and check for recent publications on your topic.

1.6 RECOGNIZE THAT PLANNING TAKES TIME AND PLANNING SAVES TIME

Sometimes, one of the most difficult things for busy residents and faculty mentors to appreciate is that the **time devoted to developing a high-quality, feasible project is time well spent**. Of course, as a busy clinician, the last thing one wants is another "time-consuming" task.

Although there are no short cuts when developing a research study, the **time spent planning reduces the overall time invested**. For some reason, people rarely believe this. The philosophy seems to be: the sooner one starts, the sooner one is done (**Box 1.3**).

Box 1.3   Why Does a Lack of Planning End Up Taking More Time?

There are several ways time is wasted when one does *not* plan sufficiently. Perhaps, after a study is approved by an ethics committee and data collection begins, the investigators realize they need additional data points. They must now submit an amendment request and wait for approval before the study continues. Perhaps, at the end of the study, an investigator discovers there are not enough subjects for statistical analysis and the work is unpublishable. The power analysis may have been skipped or done incorrectly because the investigator did not think it was necessary to consult with a statistician. Perhaps a study has the necessary subjects and data points but, when submitted for publication, it is rejected by the journal editor because the study is too similar to recently published articles. The investigator may not have done a thorough literature search before initiating the study or failed to review the latest literature before submitting to the journal.

Remember: Planning eliminates preventable events that slow or end a project's success.

Keep in mind that **time spent in the early stages saves time in the subsequent stages**. For example, taking notes while reading the literature helps you to keep track of the main points and choose citations to include in subsequent papers, proposals, or presentations. Drafting a grant application clarifies your thoughts, refines your approach, and gives you text to modify for a future manuscript.

Thus, if you **produce quality work early in the process, you will have valuable materials to reuse later**.

Every time you are tempted to just plow ahead with a project, remind yourself that the initial time devoted will pay off in the end. Consider how much time you save when you review notes compared to re-reading articles. Think about how much easier it is to revise existing text than it is to write new drafts (**Box 1.4**).

The mere thought of the effort required to initiate a new project leads some would-be investigators to give up without trying. Yes, it takes time to read literature and plan a worthwhile project, but with some **dedicated, focused time you will find** that it is **not as bad as anticipated**, especially if you **begin with a small project** that addresses a question **you have a genuine interest in answering**.

Note: **Variations of the phrase "dedicated and focused time" are repeated throughout this chapter for a reason**. Answering calls, texts, and emails is not time spent on research. No one can read or plan effectively when interrupted.

Tip: **Stay focused**. One reason why inexperienced investigators give up on research is because they have too many things going on at the same time and assume that lack of progress is due to research being too difficult or time consuming.

Hint: Take notes whenever you read the literature or discuss ideas with colleagues. With so many other responsibilities and thoughts dominating your day, it is easy to forget information you will need later. **Having good notes will make your research life much, much easier**.

Box 1.4   Faculty Perspective: What I Learned from My Mistakes

One of the first projects I started as a new faculty member was inspired by an article I read. Plans were made, Institutional Review Board (IRB) approval was obtained, the study began, and data were collected. After two to three years, there was enough data to report. However, as I prepared to write the manuscript, I realized there was no record of my original literature search, no copies of the papers read, or even the title of the article that generated the idea. **All that work had to be repeated**. Learning from this experience, as I prepared for my next study, I stored an electronic file of each article I read. As I read each article (in paper format) I made notes of salient points (electronically) and indicated how they may relate to my new study. When it came time to write the manuscript, reviewing those notes took very little time and provided the basis for the write-up.

My experiences confirmed that **time invested at the beginning of a project saves time at the end of the project**.

1.7 PLAN TO DISSEMINATE YOUR FINDINGS

Sharing your findings is part of the research process. Projects that are specific to your institution or community may be presented at lectures to colleagues or at small regional **conferences** such as a resident research day. Some projects will be of broader interest and sufficiently developed to present at larger regional, national, or international conferences. Presenting your work, even preliminary findings, is an opportunity to share your expertise, get input from others, and network with colleagues in your field. Chapters 15–17 describe how to prepare and present your work at conferences.

Publications disseminate your findings to the broadest audience, and you should begin projects with the intention of publishing your work in peer-reviewed journals. When investigators think about journals, their first thoughts are often of the prominent journals in their field. However, there are many other reputable journals, including those dedicated to medical and allied health education.

Always confirm the quality of a journal prior to submission. Never publish in "predatory" journals that accept papers without a verifiable, rigorous peer-review process (see Chapter 11, Box 11.4).

Note: Some journals include sections for resident research, essays, and perspectives.

Tip: See Chapters 10–12 on how to write and submit manuscripts to reputable journals.

Hint: **If, for any reason, your study is incomplete or your data are unreliable, do not try to publish**. It wastes your time, the reviewers' time, and the editor's time.

1.8 REMEMBER SOME OF THE KEYS TO SUCCESS

DEDICATE TIME TO THINK

You must set aside some time to think about your project. Just as you will get into the habit of setting aside dedicated time for reading, you will dedicate time to think through your project **without interruptions**. The crucial phrase is "without interruptions." Once you lose your train of thought, it takes time to get it back. Some of your thinking and planning can be done outside of an office. For many, ideas seem to flow best while running, cooking, or commuting to work. Use such times to think about your ideas, then use your dedicated office time to polish your thoughts and work through the details of your project.

PREVENT SCHOLARLY ACTIVITIES FROM FALLING TO THE END OF YOUR TO-DO LIST

There are many ways that investigators get pulled away from research, even when they are assigned time that is intended for scholarly work. It is easy to get into the mindset that "doing something," whether taking a phone call or attending a meeting, is more important than planning a project. Perhaps it is because reading and thinking appear passive and therefore expendable. **If you do not view reading and thinking as active, important activities, you will find it difficult to make progress.** Set aside time, stick to your schedule, and do not accept interruptions or changes unless there is a true emergency. You will be surprised how much you can get done when you use your reserved time for focused reading and thinking.

KEEP EVERYTHING IN PERSPECTIVE

The idea that **success begets success** applies to research. Start with something you can do, even if it is only a small pilot project that you present at a regional conference but never publish. **Any presentation of your work counts as scholarly activity and is a success.** The more experience you have in designing, completing, and summarizing findings, the easier it will be to tackle another project. **As with other areas of medicine, every experience makes subsequent efforts easier.**

BE PATIENT

It is typical to present posters at conferences for two to three years before publishing a paper. Sometimes, the presentations reflect progress on a single project; at other times, they are about unrelated projects. Experience presenting research and interacting with colleagues helps establish your credibility. **The quality of your studies and presentations are what matter.** Focus on completing ethical studies, producing trustworthy data, and discussing your work clearly and concisely.

ACCEPT THAT REJECTIONS AND REQUESTS FOR REVISIONS ARE THE NORM

A manuscript will usually be submitted more than once before it is accepted for publication; a grant application will probably be denied the first time; an ethics committee will likely request additional information before approving your study. Some of your papers and applications may be accepted on the first submission, but do not take it personally when they are not. Rejections and revisions are simply part of scholarly work. While never pleasant, they **should not discourage you from further efforts.** Talk with experienced investigators to see how they deal with rejections and how they handle suggestions from reviewers. Sometimes, reviewers make comments that are irritating or inaccurate. Sometimes, they offer helpful critiques. You need to be prepared to deal effectively with all types of feedback. Chapter 11 provides information on how to respond to manuscript reviews and Chapter 13 provides advice on how to address grant reviews.

1.9 CONCLUSIONS

For most new investigators, the most difficult part of research is getting started. It helps to acknowledge that difficulty, as it is a real hurdle which everyone faces, even experienced investigators. It is also important to recognize it is mainly a self-imposed barrier. Once you commit dedicated time and effort to developing a project, you will make progress. As you gain experience, it becomes easier to move a project to completion. The following chapters explain how to successfully initiate, complete, and disseminate your scholarly work.

Remember that the primary goal of scholarship is to disseminate quality work. Never rush to present or publish just to "get it over with" or to have something on your curriculum vitae. Colleagues, current and future, will see your work. You never want to publish something that you must later retract or admit you never understood well enough to recognize as being of poor quality.

REFERENCES AND RESOURCES

ACCREDITATION COUNCIL FOR GRADUATE MEDICAL EDUCATION (ACGME)
https://www.acgme.org

ACGME COMMON PROGRAM REQUIREMENTS
This document includes information on scholarly activity requirements for faculty and residents.
- https://www.acgme.org/Portals/0/PFAssets/ProgramRequirements/ CPRResidency2020.pdf

EDUCATION-BASED PROJECTS
Investigators interested in educational assessment and research can consult peer-reviewed publications such as:

MedEdPortal, an open access journal of teaching and learning resources in the health professions, published by the Association of American Medical Colleges (AAMC), that publishes peer-reviewed educational resources used across the health professions.
- https://www.mededportal.org

Journal of Graduate Medical Education (JGME), an open access journal from the ACGME that provides content and resources for residents and faculty interested in projects related to education and assessment. Content includes original research, educational innovations, review articles, and commentaries about graduate medical education.
- https://meridian.allenpress.com/jgme

Academic Medicine, a publication of the American Medical Association that includes articles and resources related to academic medicine, policy, education and training, research, and clinical practice.
- https://journals.lww.com/academicmedicine/pages/default.aspx

QUALITY IMPROVEMENT (QI)/QUALITY ASSURANCE (QA) PROJECTS
Investigators interested in quality improvement and patient safety projects can consult online resources and publications such as:

Agency for Healthcare Research and Quality (AHRQ). AHRQ is a United States federal agency, focused on safety and quality in American healthcare systems. Their website provides tools, publications, data resources, and other materials.
- https://www.ahrq.gov

AHRQ Quality Improvement Toolkit with Templates, Instructions, and Examples.
- https://www.ahrq.gov/evidencenow/tools/qi-essentials-toolkit.html

Quality Improvement Toolkit: Improved, Safer Care for You and Your Patients. 2019 Health Quality & Safety Commission of New Zealand.
- Falls-toolkit (hqsc.govt.nz)

Patient/Problem, Intervention, Comparison, and Outcome (PICO)

PICO Linguist (nih.gov)
- https://www.nlm.nih.gov/oet/ed/pubmed/pubmed_in_ebp/02-100.html

CLINICAL RESEARCH PROJECTS
For those interested in clinical research projects, see references and resources listed in Chapters 4–6.

CHAPTER 2

Literature Searches: Finding What Is Known and Unknown about a Topic

Lynne M. Bianchi, Ph.D., Ajaipal S. Kang, M.D., and Justin Puller, M.D.

Tips for Success:

Use more than one bibliographic database to identify relevant references. Keep track of the keywords and filters you use during every literature search.

Warning:

No single database accesses every relevant reference.

Key Concept: Bibliographic databases include features to save, sort, format, and export your references. Use the available features to save time and limit frustration.

When initiating a new project, one of your first tasks is to identify and read literature relevant to the topic of interest. Reading literature provides background knowledge, identifies unanswered questions, and helps focus your ideas into a clear and meaningful project.

To locate relevant material, you conduct a **literature search**. For basic science and clinical research projects, most of the required information will be found in research papers published in medical and science journals. Prior to the 1990s, investigators searched for journal articles using paper-based reference materials such as *Index Medicus* in university and medical libraries. Now, investigators search for literature using online **bibliographic databases** that rapidly search thousands of journals, books, and other resources at the same time. Pertinent materials are identified based on the **keywords** you enter into the database **search engine** (**Box 2.1**).

There are several bibliographic databases available, and, although some of the same materials are identified in all of them, each has its own focus, advantages, and features. This chapter outlines how to select appropriate databases and keywords to suit your needs, find relevant references outside of the databases, and save and organize selected references for future use. **Understanding how to search effectively will save time and ensure you find necessary materials**.

DOI: 10.1201/9781003126478-2

Box 2.1   Common Terms

Keywords, also called **search terms**, describe characteristics associated with an area of interest. The words may be related to the main topic, study methods, or characteristics of a study population. Any term you associate with your topic is a potential keyword.

Search engines are computer programs that locate information based on the keywords entered. They are used, for example, when entering terms to search the World Wide Web and bibliographic databases.

Bibliographic databases are searchable computer programs that identify published materials. A database returns citations and may provide links for full-text articles, books, or other materials.

Citation indices provide information about how often a reference has been cited and where it was cited. Some databases include citation indices.

Reference managers are computer programs that store, organize, and format citations. The citations may be entered manually or downloaded from a database.

2.1 CHOOSE DATABASES AND KEYWORDS THAT FIT YOUR RESEARCH GOALS

You will conduct literature searches many times throughout your career. Sometimes you will seek the latest information on **patient care**, sometimes you will review the literature to **prepare a lecture**. You must always conduct a literature search before you **begin a new study** and again when you **conclude a study**. The purpose of your literature search will influence your search methods.

SELECT BIBLIOGRAPHIC DATABASES THAT ACCESS THE INFORMATION YOU SEEK

Medically focused databases provide references from scholarly journals, books, conference proceedings, dissertations, and other sources.

The same journals are accessed by multiple databases, so you will find many of the same references in every database you use. However, each database also retrieves materials that others do not. Thus, it is always beneficial to use more than one database. You will discover **it does not take much more time to search additional databases**, especially once you are familiar with the features of each. Searching multiple databases is necessary when conducting a systematic literature review (see **Box 2.3**).

Consider what information you seek, then **choose appropriate databases**. Databases differ in their **content, search strategies, features**, and **cost**. For example, some databases are focused on research, whereas others are focused on patient care. Some only search for the terms you include, others automatically search for terms related to the keywords you enter. Some databases are free, while others require an institutional or personal subscription. **Table 2.1 lists common databases, their features, and links to frequently asked questions and online tutorials for each.**

Table 2.1 Examples of Databases and Features

Key:
Save Searches? Can users save searches to a personal database account?
Export? Can references be exported to a citation manager (software or online programs)?
Format AMA style? Can a list of citations be formatted and saved (without use of a citation manager)?
New article alerts? Can users request updates on new publications related to search terms?
ToC alerts: Users receive the table of contents from selected journals when new issues are available.
Abbreviations: AMA, American Medical Association; NLM, National Library of Medicine; ToC, Table of Contents

Databases Associated with the United States National Library of Medicine

Database	Focus	Access	Publisher	Save Searches?	Export?	Format AMA Style?	New Article Alerts?	FAQs/Tutorials
MEDLINE	Biomedical sciences, clinical sciences	Free	NLM	Yes via PubMed	Yes via PubMed	Yes via PubMed	Yes via PubMed	MEDLINE Resources: https://www.nlm.nih.gov/bsd/pmresources.html MeSH Resources: https://www.nlm.nih.gov/mesh/meshhome.html
PubMed	Biomedical sciences, clinical sciences	Free	NLM	Yes	Yes	Yes	Yes	https://pubmed.ncbi.nlm.nih.gov/help/ https://pubmed.ncbi.nlm.nih.gov/about/

Subscription Databases Focused on Biomedical Literature

Database	Focus	Access	Publisher	Save Searches?	Export?	Format AMA Style?	New Article Alerts?	FAQs/Tutorials
OVID	Biomedical sciences, clinical sciences, clinical care	Subscription	Wolter Kluwer	Yes	Yes	Yes	Yes	https://www.ovid.com/support-training/product-training/tutorials-demos.html
EMBASE	Biomedical sciences, pharmacology, toxicology	Subscription	Elsevier	Yes	Yes	Yes	Yes	https://www.elsevier.com/solutions/embase-biomedical-research/learn-and-support
Clinical Key	Medicine, nursing, pharmacy, education	Subscription	Elsevier	Yes	No	No	No; ToC alerts	https://p.widencdn.net/bmvrwt/Clinical-Key_New-Welcome https://www.elsevier.com/solutions/clinicalkey

Subscription Databases for Evidence-Based Medicine, Nursing, and Allied Health

Database	Focus	Access	Publisher	Save Searches?	Export?	Format AMA Style?	New Article Alerts?	FAQs/Tutorials
Cochrane Library	Evidence-based medicine, clinical trials	Country dependent	Wiley	Yes	Yes	No	Yes	https://www.wiley.com/network/cochranelibrary training
TRIP	Evidence-based medicine	Free and subscription versions	TRIP Database LTD	Yes	Yes (PRO)	No	Yes	https://www.tripdatabase.com/how-to-use-trip
CINAHL	Nursing, allied health, education, administration	Subscription	EBSCO Inc.	Yes	Yes	No	Yes	https://connect.ebsco.com/s/topic/0TO1H000000HHf5WAG/cinahl?language=en_US

(Continued)

Table 2.1 (Continued)   Examples of Databases and Features

Databases That Include Content from Social Sciences, Humanities, and Biomedical Sciences

Database	Focus	Access	Publisher	Save Searches?	Export?	Format AMA Style?	New Article Alerts?	FAQs/Tutorials
Web of Science	Multiple fields	Subscription	Clarivate Analytics	Yes	Yes	No	Yes	http://wokinfo.com/about/faq/
SpringerLink	Multiple fields	Subscription	Springer-Verlag	Yes	Yes	No	No; ToC alerts	https://support.springer.com/en/support/solutions/6000138290
Scopus	Multiple fields	Subscription	Elsevier	Yes	Yes	No	Yes	https://service.elsevier.com/app/overview/scopus/ https://www.elsevier.com/solutions/scopus/support
Science Direct	Multiple fields	Subscription	Elsevier	No	Yes	No	Yes	https://service.elsevier.com/app/answers/detail/a_id/10263/supporthub/sciencedirect/ https://service.elsevier.com/app/home/supporthub/sciencedirect/
Google Scholar	Multiple fields	Free	Google	Yes	Yes	No	Yes	https://scholar.google.com/intl/en/scholar/help.html#overview

One of the best-known databases, **MEDLINE**, is freely available from the United States (U.S.) National Library of Medicine (NLM). MEDLINE is easily searched using PubMed (a free search engine and biomedical/life sciences database, described below). Because the references in MEDLINE are **relevant to most biomedical fields**, several subscription databases also retrieve materials from MEDLINE. **PubMed and the subscription databases are distinguished from one another by the materials they access outside of MEDLINE.** In the descriptions that follow, MEDLINE content is explained first, followed by the unique characteristics of some other popular biomedical and healthcare-focused databases.

Note: University, medical school, and hospital libraries usually have subscriptions to at least one medically focused database. Check to see which databases you can access.

Databases Associated with the National Library of Medicine

> *MEDLINE* identifies references from over 5,000 journals and selected newsletters, magazines, and newspapers related to life, behavioral, chemical, and environmental sciences, marine and plant biology, bioengineering, and biophysics.

Most journals in MEDLINE are selected by a panel of external reviewers, the Literature Selection Technical Review Committee. Additional journals are identified by the NLM and the National Institutes of Health (NIH). All journals are reviewed annually, and titles are included or excluded based on whether they meet established criteria. Thus, a benefit of using MEDLINE is that all the **references identified come from reputable, scholarly journals**.

Another advantage of MEDLINE is that it uses consistent terms **indexed by medical subject headings (MeSH)**. MeSH terms are organized in a tree-like structure with sixteen main branches and multiple sub-branches. MeSH terms are assigned to every citation in MEDLNE using established indexing criteria. Computer-based methods and NLM indexers assign MeSH terms based on the content of an article.

Note: MEDLINE identifies citations from 1966 to the present. Articles published before 1966 are searched using OLDMEDLINE.

> *PubMed* is a free online search engine and database that accesses **MEDLINE** and other **NLM content**, including journals outside the scope of MEDLINE, articles not yet in MEDLINE, articles available online ahead of print, **books** on the National Center for Biotechnology Information (NCBI) bookshelf, and full-text, peer-reviewed articles deposited in **PubMed Central (PMC)**. PubMed has been available since 1996 and was updated to a new format in 2020.

Searches in PubMed are **designed to return the largest number of citations**. For each keyword entered, the broader MeSH term and all the associated sub-branch terms are searched using a process called **exploding**. To return fewer references, you can turn off automatic exploding or apply **filters**. For example, you may want to restrict the search to certain publication dates or study populations.

Features: PubMed provides links to many full-text articles. Icons are displayed that indicate if the full text manuscript is available from the publisher, your institution, or PMC.

PubMed includes **options for saving, exporting**, and **formatting** selected references. References can be **sorted** by date, relevancy, author, or journal. An **alerts** feature can be activated to notify you of new publications related to your search terms.

For those interested in clinical research, the **Clinical Queries** link located on the PubMed homepage under the 'Find' column (below the search box) returns references for the topic of interest under three headings at once: **clinical study categories, systematic reviews**, and **medical genetics**. Using the associated pull-down menus, you can focus on topics such as diagnosis or management.

The **MeSH Database,** located under the 'Explore' column on the PubMed homepage, provides suggestions for keywords to use in PubMed or other databases.

Note: Articles cited in PubMed receive a unique PubMed identifier (PMID).

Tip: PMIDs are included in department annual reports submitted to the accreditation council governing U.S. residency programs.

Hint: When appropriate, publish in journals cited in PubMed to ensure discoverability and a PMID for your article.

Subscription Databases Focused on Biomedical Literature

> *OVID* is a subscription database that provides links to many full-text articles and books published from 1946 to the present. OVID identifies references in **MEDLINE** but does not search other databases at the NLM. OVID does, however, include access to **EMBASE** (Exerpta Medica) and the **Cochrane Database of Systematic Reviews (CDSR)**, described below.

OVID will not automatically explode search terms, but an option to expand keywords to include related terms is available.

Features: Options for **saving, exporting,** and **formatting references** are available. An **alert** feature can be selected to receive updates when new publications are available.

The publisher offers options for those who wish to **search in Chinese, Spanish,** or **French**.

> *EMBASE* is available through OVID or as a stand-alone subscription database. EMBASE includes **additional journals** not accessed by MEDLINE or OLDMEDLINE and retrieves references for **conference abstracts**.

Articles in EMBASE are indexed using **Emtree**, a system that includes synonyms for MeSH terms and additional **terms related to drugs, pharmacology,** and **medical devices**.

Features: Users can **save, export,** and **format** selected references and receive new article **alerts**.

> *ClinicalKey* is a subscription database for references focused on clinical care. It includes specific **content targeted to physicians, nurses, pharmacists, faculty,** and **students**.

Resources include journal **articles, books, drug monographs, clinical guidelines, clinical calculators, videos,** and **patient education materials**.

Features: Search **filters** help identify relevant content within each target area and results can be **saved** and **printed**. A unique feature of ClinicalKey is the option to **incorporate images into PowerPoint slides**.

Subscription Databases for Evidence-Based Medicine, Nursing, and Allied Health

Cochrane Library is a group of databases focused on evidence-based medicine and randomized control trials (RCTs). Databases in the Cochrane Library include the **Cochrane Database of Systematic Reviews (CDSR), Cochrane Clinical Answers,** and **CENTRAL (Cochrane Central Register of Controlled Trials)**. These databases are helpful for identifying **systemic reviews** of healthcare topics, summaries of up-to-date information on **clinical care**, and **clinical trial descriptions**.

Search options include keyword, author, trial registry number, and categories listed under the pull-down menus. The **search options** allow you to focus your search on specific conditions, systems, methods, or subspecialties. **Access is free to users in countries that subscribe**, such as the United Kingdom and Denmark, and for selected **low-income countries**. Institutions in other countries, including the United States, purchase subscriptions to the Cochrane Library.

Features: Returned references can be **sorted** alphabetically, by publication date, or by relevancy. The Cochrane Library includes **save**, **export**, and article **alert** features. A **Spanish** language version is available.

The TRIP database also provides content related to **evidence-based medicine**. It pulls clinically relevant references from PubMed and other sources. The **basic version (TRIP)** is free, and an **advanced version** (TRIP PRO) is available by subscription to individuals or institutions.

Features: Search results include **icons to indicate the level of evidence** on the evidence base medicine pyramid (see, for example, Box 4.1). Results can be **sorted** by date of publication, quality of evidence, relevance, or popularity. Additional filters identify materials focused on **patient education** and **country-specific guidelines**.

TRIP PRO includes access to additional materials, videos, and medical images and features for **filtering, accessing,** and **exporting** references.

CINAHL (Cumulative Index to Nursing and Allied Health Literature) focuses on **nursing, paramedical sciences, education, behavioral sciences**, and **health administration**.

This subscription database identifies references from journals, books, pamphlets, and dissertations related to biomedical and allied health topics. CINAHL uses subject headings based on **MeSH** but also includes headings related to **nursing** and **allied health**.

Features: References can be **saved** and **exported**. **Alerts** can be activated to receive updates on publications related to selected keywords.

CINAHL includes access to available **audiovisual materials, software, research surveys**, and **questionnaires**.

Tip: If you are unsure which database to use, **start with PubMed**. Access is free, cited journals are vetted by a committee, and the literature identified is focused on biomedical topics.

Hint: If you need more information about patient care, searches in **CINAHL, TRIP**, or the **Cochrane Library** may be useful. If information on drug pharmacology or toxicology is needed, **EMBASE** might prove the most helpful. If you need information on existing research instruments, such as surveys, **CINAHL** may have the materials you seek.

Databases That Include Content Outside of Biomedical Literature

The **Web of Science, SpringerLink, Scopus**, and **Science Direct** are subscription databases that access **biomedical literature** as well as **social science and humanities journals** not accessed in other databases.

Features: Methods for **saving** and **exporting** selected search results are available in each of these databases. **Web of Science** includes an article **alert** feature.

GET ASSISTANCE USING DATABASES

When using a database for the first time, it is helpful to consult a **medical librarian**. A librarian can help identify the right databases for your needs and guide you in best practices for each.

If you do not have a librarian at your institution, assistance from a librarian at a local university or your former medical school may be available. It may also be beneficial to consult your research director, faculty mentors, or fellow residents familiar with the databases.

Much of the information you need to get started is available online. Most of the databases include **online tutorials, frequently asked questions,** and **step-by-step instructions on how to conduct and save searches** (see links in **Table 2.1**).

It is worth spending time learning about the features of the databases you use. Time spent viewing the online tutorials or getting assistance from a librarian or colleague will help you identify important features and reveal any less obvious steps to locating, sorting, saving, and exporting your references.

Remember: Bibliographic databases are designed with features that are useful to investigators. Understanding how to use those features will save you hours of work.

Tip: Many university libraries provide helpful online descriptions that highlight differences among databases, and several include tutorials on how to use them.

IDENTIFY APPROPRIATE SEARCH TERMS

The purpose of your literature search will influence your search strategies. At times, your searches will be broad, seeking as much information as you can about a topic. At other times, your searches will be narrow, focused on specific information.

To begin a literature search, think about what you want to learn, and draft a list of **keywords** or phrases associated with topics of interest. These become the **search terms** you enter in a database.

When developing your keyword list, **be sure to include variations of the word you are searching**. A given database may not recognize one of the terms and thus omit relevant references. For example, some diseases are known by more than one name (e.g., myalgic encephalomyelitis, chronic fatigue syndrome) and some originally named after a physician are now identified with a descriptive term (e.g., Wernicke's aphasia, receptive aphasia). In other instances, different words refer to the same thing (e.g., adrenaline, epinephrine).

If you need help compiling keywords, look at words in the **titles, abstracts, and keyword lists from papers** about your topic. The keyword list associated with a journal article is typically listed below the abstract. These keywords were selected by the authors to highlight content of their article and often provide ideas for search terms.

Additionally, most databases include ways to identify more keywords. For example, as you type in one keyword, related terms are suggested. A searchable **MeSH database**, available *via* PubMed, identifies keywords applicable to MEDLINE and other databases.

When developing search terms, the goal is to create a list of words that identifies as many relevant citations as possible while keeping your search focused. It is therefore helpful to **know how search terms are managed in the databases** you use. For example, some databases automatically search related terms, using the process called exploding, whereas others do not. In some databases, adding Boolean terms, such as AND or OR, expands the search, but in other databases such terms restrict the search.

No matter what keywords or Boolean terms you enter, you will get some references that are unrelated to your needs (**Box 2.2**). If you find you are getting too many citations, **refine your search using filters**. For example, you may want to limit your search by publication dates, article format (e.g., review article, clinical study, case report), subject characteristics (e.g., age, gender), or other criteria.

Tip: **MeSH on Demand**, accessed *via* PubMed, is a quick way to identify keywords to include when submitting your own manuscripts. Upload your abstract or manuscript for a list of suggested MeSH terms.

Box 2.2   Sifting through the References Identified with Your Search Terms

Any search will yield references pertinent to your goals and several that are not. For example, when searching for references about a surgical outcome known to plastic surgeons as a "dog ear deformity," some completely unrelated articles about dogs and their ears were identified. To a plastic surgeon, a dog ear deformity refers to the bunching and outward extension of tissue at the ends of an incision. Someone thought the little triangle-like shapes that extended above the incision line looked like dog ears, and that term has persisted.

A 2021 search in PubMed with the words "dog ear deformity surgery" produced 123 references. Reading through the list of references, it was apparent that 34 of the 123 were about dogs. Four were clearly about people whose ears were injured by dog bites, and 11 were about surgery on human ear deformities. Sifting through 123 references to eliminate irrelevant articles may sound a bit grueling; however, it took less than ten minutes to scan the titles and identify the ones that were obviously not about the dog ear deformity of interest. Applying a filter to limit references to those discussing humans reduced the list to 50, making it even easier to sort through the records and choose papers of interest.

Filters are especially helpful when your search terms produce thousands of references. For example, searching "ear" in PubMed returns references for any papers dealing with the outer ear, middle ear, and inner ear. PubMed automatically explodes search terms ensuring you find every reference identified with ear-related terms. A search from 2021 found nearly 200,000 references about ears. Limiting the search to the past five years left about 35,000 references. Adding a filter to include only papers about humans, reduced the titles to under 20,000. A filter to limit the search to systematic reviews about human ears published in the past five years, left 857 references. Further focusing the search on systematic reviews of human *inner* ears from the past five years left 57 references.

It takes very little time to add filters and pare down a list of references. **The key to a successful literature search is finding a balance between adding filters to focus your search without losing articles of interest**. For every search, you will experiment with combinations of keywords and filters to find the strategy right for your needs.

Hint: Every time you conduct a literature search, record the date, keyword, and filter combinations used, and the number of references returned for each. Not only will you have a record of what you searched, you will identify search strategies best suited to your needs.

2.2 NOTE ADDITIONAL WAYS TO IDENTIFY REFERENCES

CHECK RELATED ARTICLES
Most **databases** provide lists of **related articles** based on those you select. For example, PubMed provides a list of similar articles with every abstract you view. Some related articles will be included in the list generated from your original keyword search; however, additional references are also identified this way.

REVIEW REFERENCES IN PAPERS
Look at the **references which other authors cite**. You will likely find much useful material in the papers you read. However, always check databases for additional references so you are not limiting your background knowledge or biasing your interpretations based on a few authors.

Keep in mind that the references cited in a paper do not represent all the literature read by the authors, only those deemed most relevant to the content discussed.

CONSIDER MATERIALS IDENTIFIED THROUGH SEARCH ENGINES AND CITATION INDICES
Another option for locating reference materials is **Google Scholar**. This is a free, online search engine that pulls materials from a variety of online sources. Google Scholar identifies references from many scholarly journals, but also pulls citations of non-scholarly works. You will therefore **need to verify the quality and relevance of the materials**. Search filters are more limited than in databases, and references are usually sorted so those frequently and recently cited, or which offer free, full-text materials are listed first. Although Google Scholar may identify some free articles not found in databases, most people recommend Google Scholar as a supplement to academic-focused databases, but not as a primary search method.

Web of Science, Scopus, and Google Scholar include **citation indices**, measures of **how often a reference has been referenced in other publications**. Citation indices are useful for identifying references that likely represent important work in a field and may be helpful for locating landmark articles for research or teaching purposes. Many citation indices include links to papers that cite the reference of interest, providing additional material for you to consider. Although citation indices provide insight into how influential a paper is, bias occurs if they overrepresent certain authors, journals, topics, or countries.

2.3 MAKE THE MOST OF YOUR SEARCH RESULTS
It is important to keep track of **what** you searched, **where** you searched, **when** you searched, **how** you **searched,** and **what you found**.

Keeping track of your search terms and search methods is important for you, your co-investigators, and co-authors. It is important to know what has, and has not, been evaluated so efforts are not duplicated, and topics are not ignored. **Recording search strategies is also an essential step of a systematic review (Box 2.3).**

Use the article alerts feature offered by many databases to update you when new publications related to your selected search terms are available. Most databases allow you to choose how often you receive alerts and how many references to include in each update.

CINAHL, Cochrane Library, EMBASE, PubMed, OVID, SCOPUS, TRIP, and Web of Science are among the databases that offer article alerts.

Tip: To ensure broadest coverage, include alerts from **multiple databases**.

Hint: Some databases that lack article alerts offer the option to have the latest table of contents from selected journals sent to you. This is one way to keep up on findings published in journals that cover topics related to your field of study. SpringerLink and Clinical Key are among the databases that offer table of contents updates.

Maintain Good Search Records

Keep a notebook or computer file with the list of keywords you used, the date you searched, the database used, and the filters applied. The date is important, so you know when you last searched. As you progress in your project, you will conduct new searches; dating the searches allows you to focus on material published since your last search.

Save, print, and format your search results. Each of the databases mentioned in this chapter allows you to save your searches. With PubMed and most subscription databases, you can create an account to store selected references. You can also email reference lists to yourself or colleagues.

Searches can be printed, often as either a list of citations or as citations with abstracts and other identifiers, such as author affiliation, digital object identifier (doi), PMID, and keywords.

Many of the databases give you the option to **format** the references into one of the **common reference styles**, such as **AMA** (American Medical Association) and **APA** (American Psychological Association). This is extremely helpful when preparing the reference section of a manuscript, presentation, or proposal as you will not have to retype or reformat the information.

Most databases allow you to format and export references to a citation manager. Citation managers are **computer programs that store, organize, and format your references**.

Citation manager software may be purchased by individual users (e.g., **EndNote**) or accessed through an institutional subscription (e.g., **RefWorks**). Some online citation managers are free for a limited amount of storage with additional storage and features available for purchase (e.g., **Mendeley** and **Zotero**).

Citation management software may not be needed for a single project if you can collect, store, and format your references easily. **For larger projects**, such as systematic reviews or studies that will continue for multiple years, having a citation management system will be helpful.

Each citation manager has methods for organizing and retrieving your references so those related to a particular project can be quickly identified. If you are unfamiliar with citation mangers, talk with mentors or a librarian for advice on which to use.

Box 2.3   The Systematic Literature Review: Formal Search Strategies Required

A systematic review is a special type of **literature search designed to answer a clinical question**, most often related to patient care. Examples include evaluating which doses of medication effectively treat a condition or which surgical approach produces the best outcome. Systematic reviews are used as part of evidence-based medical practices because they **describe and synthesize findings from all available studies**. Some systematic reviews include **meta-analyses** in which quantitative data from each study are pooled and analyzed with appropriate statistical methods.

The goal of a systematic review is to summarize all available data and provide broad conclusions, recommendations, or algorithms that improve knowledge and patient care. Thus, appropriate and clearly defined search criteria must be used.

Two main components of a systematic review are (1) defining the **question to address** and (2) establishing the **search strategy** to find the relevant literature.

Systematic reviews involve a team of investigators who work together to define the question, establish search criteria, select appropriate databases, identify relevant studies, and summarize findings.

The investigators **first state the hypothesis or study objective**. They note what data they will seek in the literature, create a list of search terms, agree on which databases to search, and **determine criteria** to select articles relevant to the review.

Inclusion and exclusion criteria are defined prior to the literature search. Criteria for **inclusion** may be peer-reviewed research articles in languages the authors can read, publication dates, and human subjects. Some authors may accept data from prospective randomized trials, retrospective studies, observational studies, case series, and case reports. Some may exclude data from case series or case reports. **Exclusion** criteria often include review articles, recommendations, expert statements, technical reports, and animal studies.

Once search terms and eligibility criteria are agreed upon, the literature search is performed using **several databases**. To identify additional articles, investigators usually review the **reference sections** of identified articles and **manually search** any journals not included in the databases.

Because the goal is to identify all potentially relevant articles, the process begins by casting a wide net. The investigators initially review references identified in the databases to remove duplicate articles. Next, titles and abstracts are screened to select articles that appear to meet the criteria. The candidate articles are read to confirm eligibility. An investigator may read a subset of articles, or all investigators may read all candidate articles. Any conflicts regarding eligibility are resolved by a predetermined method, such as review of those articles by another investigator.

Once all eligible articles are identified, the authors organize the data from each study. Demographic information, level of evidence, and study outcomes are usually recorded. Based on the available evidence and goals of the study, a meta-analysis may be performed.

Note: A systematic review requires all search criteria to be clearly defined and adhered to throughout the process. Notes must be kept on each search. Conflicts and resolutions must be documented. These methods are included in the final manuscript so that others can understand and replicate the search strategies, if desired.

Tip: Work with a medical librarian to develop search strategies.

Hint: Before beginning a systematic review, authors should review the **Preferred Reporting Items for Systematic Reviews and Meta-analyses (PRISMA) guidelines**.

KEEP NOTES ON THE REFERENCES YOU IDENTIFY

Organize the notes you take on the papers you read. You may easily recall the first few references you read on a topic, but, **as you gather more information and projects progress, it becomes increasingly difficult to recall important details or remember where you found the information**.

Traditionally, one of the best ways to keep notes about an article was to print it out, underline key points, write comments in the margin, and file it in folder for easy access. This method still works quite well. Another option is to download an electronic copy of an article, highlight key points, make notes in comment boxes, and store in a computer file for easy access. This method also works quite well. **As with other aspects of research, it is important to develop and use a system that fits how you work**.

One of the most helpful methods for organizing materials is to create **an annotated bibliography** with the full citation, your summary of the article, and relevant notes and comments. An annotated bibliography differs from a list of titles and abstracts in that you create summaries and notes that are relevant to your objectives. **The purpose is to create a document that is useful to return to as the study progresses**.

It takes a bit more time to organize references into an annotated bibliography, but the benefits of locating pertinent information when needed makes the **initial time investment worthwhile**.

Many investigators do not create an annotated bibliography (we often do not). However, many researchers wish they had an annotated bibliography when it is time to write a manuscript, grant application, or book chapter (we often do). **An annotated bibliography does not have to be a time-consuming, formal project**. It simply needs to include information that is useful to you.

To make the most of your time:

1) Keep detailed notes on each search including date, database, keywords/search terms, filters, and results
2) Find a system that works for you (computer or paper) to keep notes on relevant sources you identify
3) Create an annotated bibliography so you can more easily search through the references you have reviewed
4) Consider use of a citation manager, especially for larger projects

Hint: Keep your notes in a location and format that you can find and decipher later. Scribbling notes in a shorthand that none of your co-authors can read is not useful. Storing notes in a paper file that you lose or on a computer you can no longer access does not help. As obvious as that sounds, notes are lost more often than one might suspect.

2.4 CONCLUSIONS

Searching for references related to your topic of interest is much easier than in past decades where a trip to the library meant hours searching through bound volumes of *Index Medicus* to find materials of interest. With online databases, investigators can search thousands of journals at once by simply typing in a few keywords. The full text of many references is also available online, providing immediate access to materials.

Each online database provides multiple features to aid in searching, sorting, saving, formatting, and exporting selected references. It is important to consider the **purpose of your literature search** and identify which **databases are most likely to access the materials** you need.

It is best to **search more than one database** to ensure you retrieve the most references related to your topic of interest. Always **keep notes on the search terms** you used and when and where you searched for references. **Organize** your saved **references** with useful **summary notes** that you can refer to later.

Better quality searches and many fewer frustrations result when you devote a bit of time to planning search strategies and organizing search results.

REFERENCES AND RESOURCES

See Table 2.1 for list of databases and websites.

CHAPTER 3

Critically Reading Research Articles: Forming Opinions and Interpreting Data

Lynne M. Bianchi, Ph.D. and James A. DeLullo, M.D.

Tips for Success:

> Reflect on the information presented in each section of the article. Assess the strengths and weaknesses of a paper and compare your interpretations to those of the authors.

Warning:

> Critical reading does not mean only finding flaws.

Key Concepts: Critical reading requires thoughtful consideration of different elements of a paper. The skills developed for critical reading will improve your writing.

Physicians often start to read scientific journals in college and continue to read science and medical literature throughout their careers. Some reading is dedicated to patient-focused literature and some to research literature. To form a meaningful opinion of any of this reading, one must critically evaluate the information presented. Unfortunately, not everyone has been taught how to assess an article and many struggle to process content effectively.

This chapter focuses on how to critically read journal articles. **Critical reading** does not mean you start with a negative attitude and search for every flaw. It means you read in **a thoughtful, reflective manner, weighing your thoughts about the study, its methods, and conclusions**. Though it helps to start out with a skeptical attitude, consideration of an article's strengths and weaknesses is essential for understanding and interpreting the data.

3.1 LEARN TO READ CRITICALLY

When readers first encounter journal articles, they often read them like reference books and assume everything presented is factual. This phase usually does not last long. By the end of college or medical school, most readers develop a more cynical attitude and begin to question whether the data support the authors'

DOI: 10.1201/9781003126478-3

interpretation. Some readers become overly skeptical, doubting everything they read. Their focus is on finding shortcomings rather than considering the meaning of the work presented. For some, this phase never ends. To them, critical reading always means finding every flaw, big or small.

Critical reading requires a balanced approach. As each section of a paper is evaluated, critical readers consider strengths and weaknesses as they ponder what the data might mean. It takes some practice to develop this balanced approach, but with some guidance you can learn to evaluate the literature thoughtfully.

Note: As mentioned in Chapter 1, active reading requires dedicated, focused time without interruptions. You can never fully process material when you are distracted.

Hint: **Active reading is required for critical reading.**

EVALUATE THE CONTENT OF EACH SECTION

Most medical and science research articles follow a standardized format: Introduction, Methods, Results, and Discussion (IMRaD). The IMRaD format is designed to help readers process information in a logical and consistent manner with certain information provided in each section of the paper (see also Chapter 11 on writing journal articles). As you read, look for the expected content and note whether the authors have omitted essential information or presented any material inconsistently.

Introduction

The Introduction presents important background information and the reasons for conducting the study. When reading the Introduction section, note the **study objective**. Consider how the authors present their **rationale** for the study. Pay attention to the **references** the authors discuss and how they describe those studies. Look at when and where the other studies were published to get a sense of how much of the literature the authors present. Do you know of other papers that should have been included? Is there published evidence that contradicts the authors' rationale for the study? Do you have any insight from your own research or clinical experience that supports the rationale? To assess the Introduction, you consider the significance of the study and whether the literature supports the need for the study.

Methods

The Methods section explains how the investigators completed the study. Think about **what was done, how it was done,** and **why it was done**. Identify strengths and weaknesses of the approach. When you identify limitations, decide how serious they are.

For **experimental studies**, assess whether the methods accurately and appropriately test the authors' hypothesis. For example, was the study population appropriate for the questions asked? Was the sample size adequate? Was there an appropriate control group? How were participants identified, recruited, and assigned to groups? How were outcomes measured? Were the measurement tools validated? What statistical analyses were used? Were they appropriate for the study questions and the type of data obtained? Even if your knowledge of statistics is limited, you should have a general impression about whether the analyses fit the study (**Box 3.1**).

For **observational studies**, identify whether descriptive or analytical methods were used, and ask questions, such as whether the sample population and sample size were appropriate for the study objective. Note how subjects were identified and enrolled. What primary and secondary outcomes were measured? How were they measured? Do the outcomes align with the goals of the study? Were potential biases or confounding variables addressed? Were the statistical analyses used appropriate for the study design and the type of data collected?

Note any information that is missing or incomplete and consider how the missing information impacts your ability to interpret the results.

Results

The Results section reports the study findings in an **impartial** manner. As you read this section, consider whether the primary outcomes reported are consistent with the objectives. Note how secondary outcomes are reported. Do the authors spend more time describing those than the primary outcome?

Are all the results presented? Did the Methods suggest other data would be included? Does it seem as if some findings are being dismissed or ignored? Why might that be?

Review the figures and tables carefully. Do the findings match what the authors report in the text? Do any of the figures appear to exaggerate findings? For example, do **graphs** suggest a large difference between groups due to the scales used? Are **images** representative of the findings, or do they appear to show atypical examples that support the authors' goals?

As you review **tables**, summarize what you see and consider whether your summary matches what the authors report.

Note: You should be able to interpret the key findings from the data presented in figures, tables, and text before reading the authors' explanations in the Discussion section.

Remember: You must understand the Methods to interpret the Results. Imagine the surprise of a colleague when it was pointed out that the study he assumed involved human subjects was done with mice. While an extreme example, it highlights how interpretation depends on knowing how data were collected.

Box 3.1   When Statistics Are Not Your Forte

Look at the study design, the outcome measures, and what the authors say about them. Overall, things should make sense.

Look at which statistical tests were used and decide if they fit the type of data collected. You might want to look at charts, such as those presented in Chapter 7 (Section 7.4) to see if the tests used match the type of data collected. If the statistical tests are not appropriate for the types of the data collected, that tells you there are problems with how the data were analyzed and interpreted.

Consider whether the authors imply that there are differences even when statistical analysis indicates there are none. For example, some authors state there were "differences between groups, but they were not significant." This just means there were no differences between groups. Similarly, some authors report differences as being "nearly significant" or "not statistically significant but showing a trend." While there are statistical tests to measure trends, unless that type of analysis was completed, the term should not be used. Whenever you encounter phrasing that signals concern, you should stop and think about the data more carefully. **Let the data tell you what is important and significant, not the authors**.

If the study used advanced statistical analyses beyond anything you can figure out on your own, look at similar studies to see what others found and ask colleagues for their opinions on the different papers. **Do not accept an author's interpretation of data simply because the analyses appear impressive**.

Discussion

In the Discussion section, the authors put the findings into context. When evaluating this section, pay attention to what the authors say about their data and how their conclusions align with the results presented. **Compare your interpretations of the data with those discussed by the authors**.

Note how the authors tie their findings to existing work. Note whether the cited references are comprehensive and up-to-date.

Consider the overall tone of the Discussion. Do the authors provide a **balanced discussion** of all findings or do they only mention some outcomes? Do they offer more than one interpretation where appropriate? Does it appear that the importance of the study is exaggerated? Are the conclusions supported by the data?

Do the authors mention **limitations** of their study? Are these the same ones you detected? Not every possible limitation will be mentioned, but important ones should be discussed.

At the end of the Discussion section, you should have better insight into the topic and the strengths and weaknesses of the study. If your interpretation of the data differs from the authors', it should be clear how they arrived at their conclusions.

Tip: When drafting your own papers, evaluate each section to make sure you have included the expected content.

CHOOSE YOUR STYLE OF CRITICAL READING

There are many approaches to reading medical and scientific literature. Different methods reflect personal preferences, though all are intended to help readers process the content in a thorough and thoughtful manner. Over time, you will adopt your own preferred methods and may incorporate some of the following common suggestions:

Scan the Article before You Read It

Read the title, look at the headings and subheadings, check what methods are used, and read the abstract. Some like to read the abstract first, some prefer to scan the content first. The goal is to **get a general sense of what the paper is about before you start reading**.

Note: You will not spoil the story if you know the ending; it helps to know what is coming so you can focus your attention and consider key points in each section.

Look at the Figures before Reading the Results

It is helpful to look at the figures *before* reading the results section. This allows you to **evaluate the findings** without influence from the authors. You may not glean everything from the figures and tables, but the data presented should leave you with some impressions.

Tip: Never skip over the figures, even when skimming an article.

Read the Sections of the Paper Out of Order

Many investigators have strong opinions about which section of the paper should be read first. There is no best way, and you may change your approach depending on the content and the purpose of reading the article. Some suggestions include:

- Read the **Methods first** or you will not be able to interpret the results.
- Read the **Results first** so you can focus on the data.

- Read the **Methods last** or read only if you are interested in the details. First, focus on the Results and how the authors explain them in the Discussion.
- Read the paper **in order**, then **review** the **Methods** and **Results** carefully.

Note: Whichever order you choose to read a paper, reflect on the content presented in each section and re-read sections as necessary.

Tip: **Take notes**. Keep track of main points in each section and jot down questions that arise. Decide whether your questions reflect weaknesses in the study, missing information, or faulty interpretation. Identify unanswered questions that suggest future projects.

Hint: You may be surprised how many times you return to some papers. You might also be surprised when you do not recall reading a paper until you see your notes on it. **Good notes help you remember what a paper is about, without having to re-evaluate it**.

Remember: **If you cite the paper, you must read it in its entirety**, in whatever order you choose. The literature is filled with papers misquoting or misrepresenting findings from another study because an author did not evaluate the full article.

3.2 DECIDE WHAT IT MEANS
After you have read a paper, pause long enough to **process what the paper said**. Form **opinions** of the study question, methods, results, and conclusions. Identify the strengths of the paper. Note the weaknesses.

Think about **future studies** that could be or should be done. Would a different approach provide important information? Are there interesting or unusual secondary findings that should be evaluated?

Consider the **larger picture** of what the data mean. For example, if the authors discuss significant differences between groups, are they talking about statistically significant or clinically significant differences? Would the conclusions from the study likely apply to other populations? If not, how difficult would it be to complete a similar study with a larger, more diverse population? How might the results differ?

It also helps to **recognize the difficulties in completing the study**. As you identify weaknesses, think about likely causes. Are there technical difficulties associated with the methods? Were there challenges to recruiting the study population? The weaknesses still exist, but it helps to ponder what it would take to get more information and, more importantly, what it would mean if we could.

Remember: If you do not pause long enough to contemplate what you read, you have not used your time wisely.

3.3 CONCLUSIONS

Critical reading involves **thoughtful consideration of the content of each section of the paper**. The goal is to reflect on what is presented, weigh the strengths and weaknesses, and compare your conclusions to those of the authors. Learning to read critically will help you write better papers as you recognize what content readers need to evaluate and interpret your findings.

REFERENCES AND RESOURCES

Durbin C.G. Jr. How to read a scientific research paper. *Respir Care*. 2009;54(10):1366–1371.

Greenhalgh T. *How to Read a Paper: The Basics of Evidence-Based Medicine and Healthcare* 6th ed. West Sussex: Wiley-Blackwell; 2019.

CHAPTER 4

Basic Research Design: Developing Research Ideas into Meaningful Projects

Lynne M. Bianchi, Ph.D., Luke J. Rosielle, Ph.D.,
Justin Puller, M.D., and Kristin Juhasz, D.O.

Tips for Success:

> Define all elements of your study before you begin.
> Identify variables you can accurately measure.
> Consult with a statistician early in the process to ensure you appropriately collect data that will answer your research question.

Warning:

> Do not begin any study with human participants until you have written approval from your Institutional Review Board (IRB) or ethics committee.

Key Concept: The time devoted to optimizing your study design is time well spent.

After you have read the literature and identified an interesting, unanswered question to address, you begin to design a study that effectively answers that question. The importance of the design phase of a research study is frequently overlooked. Too often, investigators "know" what they want to do and begin a study without considering all the components. Yet, the **research design stage is critical for the success of any research project**. Your question may be interesting and important but if you start your project with the wrong study design, the data collected will be of no value to your field.

New investigators may get lost in the jargon of study design and analysis, leading some to become frustrated and lose interest in research. Yet the research process is so much more exciting than one may think based on reading about the dangers of introducing systematic errors or failing to reject an untrue null hypothesis (a type II error). Fortunately, simply by engaging in the creative, trouble-shooting processes inherent to study design, you will naturally reduce many such errors, even when you forget what they are called.

Throughout the design phase, you and your colleagues will think of ways to address a question, identify potential problems, and develop ways to

DOI: 10.1201/9781003126478-4

offset those problems. The study design phase is a fun stage of the research process. It is part of what makes research the engaging, challenging, and creative process it is. It is a phase filled with discussions such as, "I bet we could try ...," "Yes, but if we include ...," "We do not have enough patients to do that, but if we modified ..."

Two forms of biomedical research are common during residency: basic science and clinical research. **Basic science research** focuses on pre-clinical questions, whereas **clinical research focuses** on questions related to patient care. Almost all residents engage in some form of clinical research during their training. Therefore, the focus of this chapter is on how to design clinical research studies. Elements of common study designs are introduced along with their strengths and weaknesses. Associated ethical considerations and methods of analysis are listed for each design so readers know what to anticipate when planning a project using a particular approach.

Note: Subsequent chapters will provide more information on how to identify and recruit a study population (Chapter 5), effectively collect and record data (Chapter 6), analyze data with appropriate statistical tests (Chapter 7), prepare the necessary elements of an application to an IRB (Chapter 8), and obtain informed consent from potential participants (Chapter 9).

Hint: Residents who conduct **basic science research** usually work with senior members in a laboratory to formulate questions and experimental designs consistent with the goals and resources of that lab. Basic science studies may involve animal models, cell cultures, cell lines, biospecimens, or computer modeling. These studies often seek information that will one day benefit clinical care; however, they are not intended to be of immediate clinical use and do not need to demonstrate a direct link to the clinical setting.

4.1 DECIDE HOW TO ANSWER YOUR RESEARCH QUESTION

Once you define your research question, begin to consider what information you could collect and which procedures would gather that information. This initial stage is often called **brainstorming**, the exchanges you and your colleagues have as you explore various ways to answer your research question.

When generating these first ideas, it is best to consider all approaches, even those beyond your resources. You will ultimately focus your ideas into a feasible project that you can complete. However, it is helpful to first consider as many alternative approaches as you can. Although you may not be able to do everything you would like, by exploring different options you ultimately develop a stronger project.

You can ask and answer questions as they arise, then rephrase them and think about them, using study design terminology and methodology, as in **Table 4.1**.

Table 4.1 Questions to Address When Developing a Study: (A) Basic questions can be answered during initial planning stages. Those questions can then be rephrased and answered using study design terminology (B).

A. Basic questions:	B. Questions phrased in study design terminology:
What do I want to know? For example, is a given treatment good for patients with a specific condition?	What are your study goals or objectives? What is your hypothesis?
What would I need to observe or measure? What data would I collect to determine if the treatment was good for those patients?	What are your independent and dependent variables? What exposures and outcomes are you going to monitor? What is your primary outcome measure? Are there secondary outcome measures?
How could I make those observations or measurements? What information do I need to collect? How will I get that information from participants?	What levels of measurement are you using (continuous, dichotomous, ordinal, or nominal)?
How could I figure that out? What ways could I test if that treatment is good for patients with that condition? Who would I need to study?	What methods will be used for data collection? Will you use an observational or experimental approach? What is your sample population? How will you recruit, select, and allocate participants?
How could I make sure I am only observing/measuring what I intend to observe/measure? What additional information might be collected that clarifies or confuses my interpretation of the answer?	What confounding variables do you need to consider? What biases could arise?
How will I know if my answer is correct? How do I know that the data I collect is an accurate reflection of the individuals and treatment I am studying?	What statistical tests are appropriate for your study design, population, and variables?

TAKE THE FIRST STEPS: SELECT A GENERAL STUDY APPROACH AND IDENTIFY MEASURABLE VARIABLES

Early in the process, you choose a general approach suitable for answering your question. For example, you decide between an observational or experimental study design and retrospective or prospective data collection.

With **observational** methods, the investigator observes what **naturally occurs** and provides a summary of findings, typically in a narrative format with quantified information included where appropriate. Analytical observational studies can also test hypotheses. **Experimental** studies involve **investigator-controlled interventions**, modifications that are manipulated and measured to determine their effects. With experimental studies, hypotheses are tested.

Retrospective studies evaluate what happened in the **past**. Questions are answered with available data, such as information found in patients' medical records. In contrast, **prospective studies** evaluate what occurs in the **future**. You collect data as it occurs naturally (observational) or in response to a change you make (experimental).

Your study approach is further shaped by who and what you choose to measure.

Who you study becomes your **study population,** the group of individuals selected to represent all the people with the characteristics of interest. The study population must be **representative of the intended target population**. You therefore carefully consider those characteristics that must be present in participants (**inclusion criteria**) and any characteristics that cannot be present (**exclusion criteria**).

What you study are called the **variables**, which are those properties that change during your study. The **independent variables** (also called predictor variables) are the properties thought to cause a change in other variables. In clinical research these are usually called **exposures, treatments,** or **risk factors**.

Dependent variables result from changes to an independent variable. These are the properties observed or measured in your study. They are also called **outcomes** or **diseases** in clinical research.

The purpose of research is to discover if changes in an independent variable (e.g., the doses of a drug or the length of exposure to a risk factor) are associated with changes in a dependent variable (e.g., the length of hospitalization or the frequency of a cancer diagnosis). Choosing appropriate, measurable variables is therefore essential for the success of a project.

CHOOSE CATEGORICAL OR CONTINUOUS VARIABLES

Independent and dependent variables are each divided into two broad categories: categorical and continuous variables.

Categorical Variables are those that have a finite number of groups or categories. Variables that can be placed into groups without any intrinsic order or ranking are called **nominal variables**; nominal variables that comprise only two categories (yes/no; right/left) are called **dichotomous** (or **binary**) variables. Variables that can be ordered or ranked in some fashion are called **ordinal** variables.

Categorical variables may be recorded with **qualitative** or **quantitative** terms. However, when numbers are assigned to nominal variables, they are usually arbitrary. For example, when collecting data, your team may choose to code "left-handed" as "1" and "right-handed" as "2". This does not imply anything about the relative value of left-handedness or right-handedness. There is nothing bigger or greater about a "right-handed" participant than a "left-handed" participant. You could just as easily assign 20 for left-handed and 30 for right-handed. Coding dichotomous variables, typically as 1, 2 or 0, 1, is done out of convention and simplicity, not to indicate value or meaning for the numbers.

Ordinal values are often seen in scales such as those to rank a patient's perceived level of pain on a scale of 0 (no pain) to 10 (worst imaginable pain). Other examples include stages of a disease (Stage I to Stage IV) and body mass index (BMI) category (e.g., 1, underweight; 2, normal; 3, overweight; 4, obese).

Although **ordinal variables** can be ranked, there is **no absolute numeric value** associated with them, only the **relative rankings**. For example, a pain score of 4 cannot be judged to be twice as painful as a score of 2; all we can say is that a score of 2 is "less painful" than a score of 4. Note that, with ordinal variables, you do not know how much of a difference there is between members of the different groups, only that one group has more or less of the variable in question. Thus, ordinal variables **lack** a property called **equal intervals**. For example, ordinal variables provide no information about the difference in weight in kilograms between one participant who is ranked as "1, underweight" and another who is ranked as "2, normal". Furthermore, the differences may vary depending on the particular "underweight" and "normal" participants you compare.

Continuous Variables, in contrast to categorical variables, have **a meaningful numeric value** that can be ordered in some way. Thus, the numbers assigned to continuous variables are **not arbitrary**.

Interval variables are measured along a continuum and therefore have the **equal intervals** property (hence the term "interval" variable). However, interval variables **lack a meaningful zero point**. Examples of interval variables are IQ scores, pH value, and temperature in degrees Celsius or Fahrenheit. There is no 0 measurement that equals no intelligence, no pH, or no heat on these scales. There is still heat at zero degrees Celsius or Fahrenheit, although it may not feel like it.

What makes interval variables different from ordinal variables is the property of equal intervals. For example, the difference between 50° and 60° Fahrenheit is the same as the difference between 30° and 40° Fahrenheit; both differ by 10 degrees. However, as with ordinal variables, multiplicative statements cannot be made about interval variables; a person with an IQ of 100 is not twice as intelligent as a person with an IQ of 50.

Ratio variables are those that have a **true 0 value**, which indicates a complete absence of that variable. Temperature on the Kelvin scale is a ratio variable because 0° Kelvin represents the complete absence of heat, a term called absolute zero (equivalent to −273.15° Celsius). Other examples of ratio variables are income, time, and weight. You can have an income of 0 (an absence of money), 0 minutes left to submit a grant application (an absence of remaining time), and after you step off a scale, the reading returns to 0, indicating an absence of weight.

Note: Ordinal data, such as those obtained from a Likert scale (e.g., a scale that ranges from "1, Strongly Agree" to "5, Strongly Disagree"; pain scale 0–10), are often treated as interval variables for statistical purposes. However, consultation with a statistician is recommended to ensure your data are collected and analyzed correctly.

SELECT LEVELS OF MEASUREMENT THAT PROVIDE THE MOST INFORMATION

When designing your study, think about which variables should be measured. In some cases, you are limited by the question asked. If you want to compare test scores in those who are left-handed with those who are right-handed, your independent variable is necessarily a categorical variable (handedness). In other cases, you can choose the type of variable to measure (ordinal, interval, ratio). Your independent variable may be from one category (categorical or continuous) and your dependent variable from another.

Choosing the variables to measure becomes an important element of your study design because the types of variables you include, called your **levels of measurement** or scales of measurement, **determine which statistical tests can be used for data analysis**. Without proper planning, you might choose an inappropriate scale of measurement and inadvertently limit the kinds of data analysis that can be done.

It is typically best to **measure variables using the highest scale of measurement possible**. For example, ratio numbers contain more information than interval numbers, which contain more information than ordinal numbers. In addition to the increased information, choosing the highest scale of measurement allows you to later convert your data to a lower scale of measurement, if desired. However, rarely, if ever, can you convert data to a higher scale of measurement. For example, if you collect the calculated BMI from each participant (ratio) you can later convert that to a BMI category (ordinal) if you decided it makes sense to summarize your data that way. However, if you only record the BMI category for each participant, there is no way to convert that back to the participant's exact BMI (ratio value). Thus, it is best to record the actual BMI rather than the BMI category.

IDENTIFY PRIMARY AND SECONDARY OUTCOME MEASURES

Every study has a **primary outcome** measure, namely the dependent variable most important for answering your research question. It may also have **secondary outcomes**, which are additional findings collected as part of the study.

Every study needs a primary outcome measure, but secondary outcome measures are optional. For example, in a study designed to assess the effectiveness of a weight loss drug, the primary outcome is the change in body weight. Blood pressure may be included as a secondary outcome measure. A lower blood pressure may be linked to an observed weight loss, or the medication may influence blood pressure directly. Additional studies are usually necessary to confirm any relationship between the independent variable and secondary outcome measures.

It is also imperative that an investigator does *not* use a secondary outcome as an alternative primary outcome. When a primary outcome is not as impressive (statistically significant) as the investigators envisioned, some are tempted to find other differences between the groups studied. This is often called a "statistical fishing expedition" because the investigators go through the data searching ("fishing") for any statistically significant outcome (see also Chapter 7). However, a study is designed to assess the primary outcome, not draw conclusions about secondary outcomes. A study investigating whether a drug promotes weight loss might include the secondary outcome measures of blood pressure, cholesterol levels, and patient-rated fatigue. If there is no statistically significant difference in weight loss (the primary outcome measure) between the treated and untreated groups, but there is a difference in blood pressure, the investigators cannot write up the results as if changes in blood pressure were the focus of the study. Instead, the study would report no difference in the primary outcome (weight loss), then present the results of the secondary outcome measures and discuss what the decreased blood pressure may mean. Another study, by the same or different investigators, could then test whether the medication lowers blood pressure.

Remember: All outcomes are identified *before* the study begins.

Tip: Always spend time considering what your measurements *cannot* tell you. Your data will provide information that helps address a gap in knowledge, but they will not reveal everything. Recognizing the limits of your measurements will make your interpretations more meaningful.

CONSIDER MEASURES THAT MIGHT CONFUSE THE RESULTS
Although you choose your independent and dependent variables, there are usually other variables that influence your outcomes. A **confounding variable**, or **confounder**, is an extraneous variable that interacts with the independent variable or affects the outcome (dependent variable). An often-cited example is the erroneous association of lung cancer, the primary outcome measure, with coffee drinking. Based on data it appears that coffee drinkers have higher rates of lung cancer than non-coffee drinkers. However, most coffee drinkers who had lung cancer also smoked cigarettes. The two habits tended to go together; the individuals often smoked while drinking coffee. In this example, coffee drinking is a confounding variable. Smoking cigarettes is the independent variable (exposure) associated with lung cancer (outcome).

It is to your advantage to **identify any obviously confounding variables prior to the start of data collection**, and then to **measure those variables during data collection**. In the example above, if we record each participant's coffee consumption, cigarette smoking, and whether they have lung cancer, we can determine the unique contributions of coffee and cigarette smoking to lung cancer rates.

It is important to note that **confounding variables can usually be dealt with *if* you measure them**, hence the importance of identifying confounding variables during the design phase of your research. Advanced statistical techniques, principally analysis of covariance (ANCOVA) and multiple regression, can factor out the effect of a confounding variable on the outcome, but only if the confounding variable has been measured.

For example, if you never thought to measure cigarette smoking in the first place, it would be impossible to determine whether cigarette smoking was or was not likely to be associated with coffee drinking or lung cancer. **Being well versed in research related to your topic is the best way to identify potential confounders**.

The accuracy of your data collection and analysis will be further complicated by biases. **Biases are defined as errors in measurement that occur consistently** and **promote one response or outcome over others**. There are over 40 forms of research biases, many of which result from **investigator** or **participant behavior, the design of a measurement tool**, or in the **way a tool is used**.

Although biases are often unintentional and unrecognized, good study design considers where biases might occur and enacts ways to minimize them. Chapters 5 and 6 further discuss different types of bias and ways to reduce their effects during participant selection and data collection.

Note: The study design phase is fluid in the beginning. You need time to refine your ideas as you consider what information is needed to answer your research question. You do not design your study in one day then go with your first plan. You rule out approaches and measurements that would not be practical for you to use and consider potential weaknesses in the approaches you can use. You may even need to modify your design shortly after data collection begins if obvious problems emerge.

Remember: The more issues you identify and address upfront, the stronger your study will be.

4.2 SELECT THE STUDY DESIGN THAT BEST ANSWERS YOUR RESEARCH QUESTION

Study designs commonly used in medically focused clinical research are described below. At times, the optimal design for your study question may not be feasible given your resources, accessible populations, and available time.

However, always **design the most thorough, highest-quality study possible**. Avoid the temptation to pick the easiest approach. Always develop a study that will provide useful information to your field.

Note: Ethical considerations are included below to remind you of key considerations for protecting participants' rights and when to contact your IRB or ethics committee. Chapters 8 and 9 describe specific procedures to follow.

Tip: If you are using a study design for the first time, consult with experienced mentors and refer to books that describe research methods in more detail before you begin. See examples in References and Resources listed at the end of this chapter.

Hint: Find a published report on a similar topic using the study design of interest, then emulate the methodology as closely as possible. Remember, the Methods section of a manuscript is purposely written with a level of detail so that other researchers could replicate the study. Thus, published reports can provide a template to follow.

Remember: Having a plan in your mind is not sufficient. You must have a detailed written study protocol. The study protocol provides structure to your project, serves as the instruction manual to guide the study team, and provides the information needed to replicate or extend your findings.

OBSERVATIONAL STUDIES: DESCRIPTIVE AND ANALYTICAL APPROACHES
Observational research is used in many disciplines. In medical research, **descriptive** and **analytical** observational approaches are common (**Figure 4.1**). For all observational studies, investigators report what **occurs naturally**; there are **no investigator interventions**. However, descriptive and analytical observational studies differ in the types of questions asked, the types of data collected, and how data are analyzed. Examples of different observational study designs are described below.

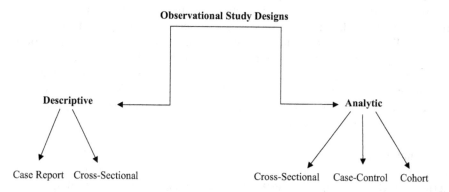

Figure 4.1   Observational study designs are either descriptive studies that lack a control group or analytic studies that include a control group.

Descriptive Observational Studies

These seek to answer questions such as **who? what? where? when?** These studies collect qualitative data, and sometimes quantitative data, about a disease, condition, or treatment. There is **no control group**. Examples of descriptive observational studies include **case studies** and **cross-sectional studies**.

Case Studies

There are two forms of case studies: case reports and case series. A **case report** describes a single patient. A **case series** describes a small number of patients. Both are used to convey information related to patient demographics, differential diagnosis, treatment, and follow-up. Case studies **do not include a control group** because they only present observations about the cases encountered. Their purpose is to share information helpful to other health care providers. These studies often note what to watch for, what to do, or what to avoid when treating similar patients.

Examples:

1) A *case report* that describes a patient presenting to the emergency department with symptoms suggestive of a benign condition that is found to be a rare but serious condition. The case details the laboratory and imaging results used to differentiate the benign from the serious condition and describes a successful treatment approach. The case gives helpful information for clinicians who encounter similar patients.

2) A *case series* that describes the clinical history, presenting symptoms, and radiographic findings of 3 patients with persistent lung damage 18 months after a viral infection. The cases alert others about potential long-term health problems in patients exposed to that virus and motivate additional studies of the long-term consequences of the virus.

Ethical considerations and requirements: Patient privacy and confidentiality are import considerations given the detailed health and demographic information provided in a case report or case series. Investigators need to remove all identifying information from any images and must be careful not to describe personal information that would lead others to identify the subject. Some institutions require IRB review and approval before beginning case studies, whereas others only require IRB review for projects describing four or more patients. Investigators must always check their institutional requirements prior to beginning a case report or case series.

Note that **patient consent** is usually needed. Many institutions and most journals require written consent from all patients described in a case report or case series. **CARE** (*Case report*) **guidelines**, referenced at the end of this chapter, should always be followed for all case studies.

Statistical analysis: Because case studies describe only a single patient or a small group of patients, statistical analysis is limited. There is no control group, and no hypotheses are tested. **Descriptive statistics** may be used to summarize quantitative findings where applicable.

Strengths: Case reports and case series are among the easiest studies to conduct because subjects are encountered and **data are collected during standard medical care**. Although authors of a case series identify patients with similar traits, they do not recruit patients: all patients are observed during regular medical practices. There are **no costs** associated with the research itself and the **time to complete is short compared with other studies**. Time is needed to gather data from the medical record, review the literature, prepare images, and write the manuscript.

Some case reports and case series are the first to describe a new disease or treatment and lead to major advances in the medical field. The first descriptions of patients with the disease ultimately identified as HIV/AIDS is a frequently cited example of how case reports lead to the identification of an emerging disease. Similarly, some of the earliest descriptions of symptoms and treatment approaches for the novel coronavirus disease 2019 (COVID-19) were found in case reports and case series. Early case reports on HIV/AIDS and COVID-19 led to large-scale studies that revealed underlying mechanisms and treatments for these diseases. Thus, case studies often serve as the starting point for further research.

Although most case studies do not have the same impact as these examples, they are still important contributions to the medical literature. Case studies are **used in medical education** and often **provide important examples of differential diagnosis** and **treatment options**. Case studies may also provide counterexamples to established theories or practices, or may document rare or unusual examples.

Limitations: Case reports and case series provide information about a single patient or small group of patients and therefore have **limited generalizability**. Because observations from one or a few patients are not enough to sway clinical practice, these studies are ranked near the bottom of the **evidence-based pyramid**, a system for ranking the value of study designs in clinical decision making (**Box 4.1**). Furthermore, the quality of these studies is often inconsistent. Some authors view case reports as an "easy" publication and put little thought into the content, purpose, or value of adding the case to the medical literature.

Note: Case reports and case series are a common form of publication for many residents and are discussed further in Chapter 12.

Tip: Rather than rush to publish for the sake of publishing, take the time to identify cases that are truly worthy of sharing and **write a report that provides information useful to other busy clinicians**.

Hint: When seeking ideas for a new project, look at case studies for topics needing further investigation.

Descriptive Cross-Sectional Studies

These studies examine participants at a **single time**. Thus, the exposure/risk factor (independent variable) is evaluated at the same time as the outcome/disease (dependent variable). **Participants are evaluated only once, there is no follow-up,** and as with other observational studies, there is **no control group.** The single time point studied may be a day, a week, or even a few months. The key is that the time is limited and defined.

Examples:

  1) A study that looks at the number of students at a single high school with nasal congestion who used electronic cigarettes during the past 48 hours.

  2) A study of the number of people born in a geographic region between 1995 and 2015 who were diagnosed with autism and breast fed for at least 4 months.

Ethical considerations and requirements: IRB consultation will be required for these studies. Depending on the details of the study, the exempt, expedited, or full committee review process will be used (see Chapter 8). If information is de-identified, so that it is not possible to link subject information to an individual, an observational cross-sectional study may qualify for exemption from IRB oversight. Investigators will need to submit a request for exemption to their IRB and wait for written IRB confirmation that the study is exempt prior to beginning the study. If it is possible to link the data to an individual, the expediated or full committee process will be used.

Whatever the method of IRB review, investigators will indicate how patient information will be protected and stored, and list who will have access to the data. Methods of obtaining informed consent (see Chapter 9) will be included, if applicable.

Investigators should follow **STROBE** (*St*rengthening the *r*eporting of *ob*servational studies in *e*pidemiology) **guidelines,** listed at the end of this chapter, when designing and reporting cross-sectional studies.

Statistical analysis: Descriptive cross-sectional studies often provide information on the **prevalence** of a disease or condition. Prevalence is an indication of **the frequency of an outcome in a population.** As with other observational studies, **descriptive statistics** may be used to summarize the data.

Strengths: Because patient outcomes are assessed at the same time as the exposure/risk factor, descriptive cross-sectional studies **provide information**

quickly and usually at a **low cost.** This approach is also useful for gathering **preliminary data** to see whether larger, more resource-intensive studies are justified.

Limitations: Descriptive cross-sectional studies **do not indicate cause or effect** because all variables are measured at the same time. For example, a diagnosis of autism among a group of students who were breast fed as infants does not indicate that breast feeding caused the autism. Conversely, finding only a few students diagnosed with autism in the breast-fed group would not indicate that breast feeding prevented autism. The study could only indicate how prevalent autism is in that sample population. Additional studies using other methods would be needed to determine if there was a cause-and-effect relationship between two variables. These studies are ranked near the bottom of the evidence-based pyramid (**Box 4.1**).

Box 4.1   Evidence-Based Medicine Uses Research Findings to Guide Clinical Practice

To help clinicians rate the quality of different studies, **evidence-based pyramids** were developed. The level of evidence is often referred to when ranking a study design. The top of the pyramid (level 1) represents those study designs most likely to provide information useful for making decisions about patient care. The bottom of the pyramid (levels 5–7, depending on the pyramid) indicates those study designs which are least likely to provide data directly applicable to clinical practice (Figure 4.2). A study at the bottom of the pyramid does not mean it lacks any valuable information; it simply indicates that those findings alone are insufficient for making clinical decisions.

The pyramid was developed in part to steer clinicians away from the long-held practices of following advice because it came from an "expert" or using an approach simply because it was common.

Although there are variations in the evidence-based pyramid, most include 5–7 levels and all place systematic reviews with meta-analyses at the top. These studies are at the top of the pyramid because they evaluate and summarize the quality of published, randomized, controlled clinical trials (see Chapter 2) and therefore are thought to provide relevant summaries for clinical decision making. Randomized, controlled trials are usually placed next and may be considered level 1 or level 2 evidence, depending in part on the quality of the trial and the number of participants who completed the study.

Experimental studies, including non-randomized, controlled trials, are always placed higher than observational studies, and observational studies without a control group are placed lower than those with a control group. Expert opinions and editorials are placed at the base of the pyramid, at the lowest level.

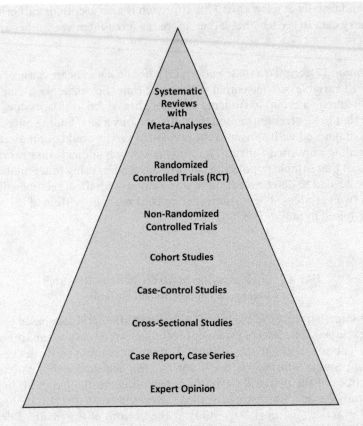

Figure 4.2   An example of an evidence-based pyramid. Evidence-based pyramids are used in ranking the relevance of study designs in guiding decisions about patient care. Those listed at or near the base of the pyramid are considered least likely to provide sufficient data for making clinical decisions. Those at or near the peak of the pyramid are more likely to provide data that directly aid clinical decision making.

Analytical Observational Studies

These studies seek to answer **why?** Unlike descriptive observational studies, analytical observational studies **include a control group**. These studies can therefore test hypotheses and be analyzed using inferential statistics. Common forms of analytical observational studies include **cross-sectional**, **case-control**, and **cohort studies**.

Analytical Cross-Sectional Studies

Like the descriptive cross-sectional studies described above, these studies focus on a **single time**, and have no follow-up. However, *analytical* cross-sectional studies **include a control group** and therefore differences between those who have the exposure or outcome of interest can be compared with those who do not. **Associations between an exposure/risk factor** and an **outcome/disease** may be identified. Because analytical cross-sectional studies include a control group, they are placed nearer the middle of the evidence-based pyramid (**Box 4.1**).

Examples:

1) A study investigating the possible association between agricultural pesticides and skin cancer. The number of farmers in a county with stage IV skin cancer who lived within 500 feet of soybean fields sprayed annually with the same pesticide for the past 15 years is compared to the number of farmers who lived within 500 feet of soybean fields that were not sprayed with that pesticide during the past 15 years.

2) A study evaluating a potential link between electronic cigarette use and nasal congestion in teenagers. Nasal congestion of at least 7 days duration is compared between a group of teenagers who has used electronic cigarettes weekly for at least 6 months and a group of teenagers who has never used electronic cigarettes.

Ethical considerations and requirements: Most analytical cross-sectional studies will require approval from an IRB *via* expedited or full committee review. Methods for protecting participant data will need to be explained in all applications. For some studies, investigators will describe how participants will be identified and recruited, and how informed consent will be obtained. **STROBE guidelines** are followed.

Statistical analysis: Data are typically analyzed using **inferential statistics** that allow the investigator to formally test a hypothesis and make comparisons between groups. The statistical tests used will be determined by the types of measurements made (categorical, continuous) and the number of groups in the study. For example, when the data from each group have a **normal distribution** and the **variables** measured are **continuous** (interval, ratio) then **parametric tests,** such as **Student's *t* test, Pearson's correlation coefficient**, or **analysis of variance (ANOVA)**, might be used. When the data are **not normally distributed** or the variables are **categorical** (nominal, ordinal), then an appropriate **non-parametric test** will be used, such as the **Chi-squared test, Fisher's exact test, Spearman's rank correlation coefficient**, or **Mann-Whitney *U* test**.

Analytical cross-sectional studies may also provide an **odds ratio**, representing the **chance an outcome will occur from a given exposure**.

Strengths: An advantage of analytical cross-sectional studies is that **multiple outcomes can be studied at one time**. Furthermore, the studies are **relatively quick** and **less expensive** than other analytical designs.

Analytical cross-sectional studies can provide information about the **status of a disease/outcome in a population** and the **association between an exposure and an outcome**. They may also indicate the **chances of developing an outcome** from a given exposure (the odds ratio).

Limitations: This design is **not appropriate** for studying **rare conditions** because it is unlikely to identify enough subjects in a population at any given time. For example, if the incidence of stage IV skin cancer is very low in the population studied, it would not be possible to identify and enroll enough participants with the disease.

Although analytical cross-sectional studies identify associations between variables, they **do not determine cause and effect** because, like the example with coffee smoking and lung cancer above, they cannot rule out all possible confounding variables. In some instances, a logical order is suggested. For example, it makes sense that smoking causes lung cancer, but not that lung cancer causes smoking. However, in other cases, it is not possible to know which came first. This is known as the **directionality problem**. For some relationships, it is impossible to determine which variable is the cause and which variable is the effect without further study. For example, living near a noisy airport may cause mental health issues. Alternatively, those who live near the airport may have pre-existing mental health issues that limit their employment and housing options. Thus, additional studies would be needed to identify the exposure/ risk factor (e.g., living near noise or mental health issues) and the outcome (e.g., living near noise or mental health issues).

Analytical cross-sectional studies are also subject to biases including **selection bias** and **recall bias.** For example, farmers whose fields were not sprayed with the pesticide may have other behaviors that limit their likelihood of developing skin cancer (membership bias, a form of selection bias). Other farmers may not recall which pesticides were used in the past 15 years (recall bias). These examples further illustrate why you cannot infer causality from an analytical cross-sectional study. It is simply impossible to rule out all biases that could explain your results.

Note: The key differences between descriptive and analytical cross-sectional studies are:

- **Descriptive** cross-sectional studies indicate **prevalence** of a disease or condition at a given time and do not include a control group.
- **Analytical** cross-sectional studies include a **control group**, provide insight into **associations**, and may indicate an **odds ratio.**

Case-Control Studies

These are another type of analytical observational study, comparing two groups: one with an outcome of interest and one without that outcome. Thus, for these studies, the **outcome** (disease or condition) is **identified first**. Individuals in the **case** group have the disease or condition while those in the **control** group do not. Investigators identify specific characteristics (e.g., risk factors) they suspect are related to the outcome and then compare the two groups to see if any characteristics are associated with either group. Case-control studies are ranked near the middle of the evidence-based pyramid (**Box 4.1**).

Case-control studies are either **retrospective** (looking at past exposures/risk factors) to identify **prevalence**, or **concurrent** (current exposures/risk factors) to identify **incidence**.

To produce the most useful data, the two groups are matched as closely as possible. Thus, cases should be representative of the population of interest and controls should be at risk of developing the disease or condition. Cases should be randomly selected, if possible. As a general guideline, investigators are advised to enroll two to four controls for every case, as previous research has noted an equal number of cases and controls is unnecessary.

Example:

> A study of beverage consumption (exposure/risk factor) and stroke (outcome) in patients admitted to a single hospital during a 6-month period. The consumption of selected beverages (green tea, orange juice, caffeinated coffee, or red wine) is compared in those admitted for stroke (cases) to those admitted for unrelated reasons with no history of stroke (controls). The investigators want to know if any of the beverages were consumed more often by either the cases or the controls.

Ethical considerations and requirements: Case-control studies will likely require approval from the IRB *via* expedited or full committee review because it is unlikely that participant information can remain de-identified throughout the data collection process. Methods for identifying cases and controls will be explained and the procedures for protecting participant privacy and confidentiality will be detailed. Patient consent may not be required if reviewing existing charts, but if investigators must contact patients, informed consent will be required. **STROBE guidelines** are followed for case-control studies.

Statistical analysis: **Inferential statistics** are typically used to compare groups. The data may reveal the **odds ratio**, the chances of developing the outcome from a given exposure, or the **relative risk**, the probability of an outcome occurring in one group compared to the probability in another.

Strengths: Case-control studies are **relatively quick** and easy to conduct and there is **no follow-up**. Additionally, this design is helpful for studying **rare outcomes** because the cases are identified in advance.

Limitations: Case-control studies can only identify potential links but **cannot determine cause and effect**. In some studies, it may be difficult to identify an appropriate control group if a variable is uncommon. For example, investigators studying the use of social media and length of hospital stay might find it difficult to identify enough patients who do not use social media. Furthermore, this approach is **not helpful** for studying cases caused by **rare exposures/risk factors** due to the difficulty of finding enough cases. In the example evaluating beverages consumed, if few participants drank green tea (rare exposure), it would not be possible to determine its influence on health outcomes.

These studies are also susceptible to biases such as **recall bias**, **reporting bias**, and **selection bias**. In the beverage study, patients may not accurately recall the volume or frequency of beverage consumption (recall bias), some may be reluctant to admit how much they consumed if they believe the behavior contributed to their medical condition (reporting bias), or the target population may not be represented if cases were enrolled from a hospital that specializes in stroke care. In this case, the study population may be skewed to those with more serious outcomes rather than representing typical patients who have had a stroke (selection bias).

Cohort Studies

These studies seek **links between an exposure and an outcome**. The **cohort** is a group of individuals with a shared characteristic such as a common risk factor, treatment, or environment. In some studies, the cohort has a shared outcome. Both prospective and retrospective cohort studies are used to identify possible causes of an outcome, though prospective cohort studies are more common.

> *Prospective cohort studies* identify a population of interest, and then follow that population over time to see who develops the outcome of interest. These are **longitudinal studies** and often take place over several years. A famous example is the Framingham Heart Study which began surveying residents (the cohort) of Framingham, Massachusetts in 1948 to identify risk factors for heart disease (outcome).

> *Retrospective cohort studies* are conducted when the exposure and outcome have already occurred. A cohort is selected based on a shared characteristic, often a particular exposure or risk factor. Records are then reviewed to identify when exposures occurred to see if there is a likely association between the exposure and an outcome. Retrospective cohort studies differ from case-control studies in that exposure status, rather than disease status, is typically the starting point.

Unlike other observational studies, **cohort studies suggest, but do not conclusively establish, a cause-and-effect relationship**. Cause and effect is supported by the temporal relationship between the exposure and the outcome. Among observational studies, cohort studies are ranked closest to the top of the evidence-based pyramid. Prospective cohort studies are placed higher on the pyramid than retrospective cohort studies.

Examples:

1) Investigators conduct a **prospective cohort study** to see if participation in team sports prior to age 50 protects older adults from health conditions commonly associated with aging. They identify a cohort of young adults between the ages of 25 and 30 who play recreational sports in three communities across New Jersey and survey the participants every 5 years to monitor health status.

2) An investigator completes a **retrospective cohort study** of a group of patients from a geographical region (risk factor) with a high prevalence of leukemia (outcome). Records are reviewed to identify risk factors/ exposures, such as length of time living in the area and proximity of one's home to a former waste disposal site.

Ethical considerations and requirements: Prospective and retrospective cohort studies are reviewed by the IRB. Because investigators access patients' health records and personal information, often over a long period of time, details explaining how confidentiality will be maintained throughout the course of the study will be important. Methods explaining recruitment and informed consent procedures will be required for any study in which patient contact occurs. Longitudinal studies also require procedures for participants to indicate ongoing consent. As with other observational research studies, **STROBE guidelines** are followed.

Statistical analysis: Cohort studies are typically evaluated with **inferential statistics to test hypotheses**, with the specific tests determined by the types of variables (categorical, continuous). Cohort studies may provide a measure of the **relative risk** of an outcome in one group *versus* another, or of **absolute risk**, the **odds of an outcome occurring during a defined period.**

Prospective studies can also determine **incidence, the number of *new* cases per specified time.**

Strengths: Cohort studies can assess one exposure and **multiple outcomes** and identify outcomes from **rare exposures**.

With **prospective cohort studies**, the outcome has not yet occurred so investigators can determine a **temporal relationship** between an exposure and outcome and **suggest causality**.

Retrospective cohort studies, like other retrospective studies, are **relatively fast** and **inexpensive** to complete.

Limitations: Cohort studies are **not appropriate** for studying **rare outcomes** because there will not be enough participants to follow. Cohort studies can only evaluate the exposures/risk factors identified at the beginning of the study. Cohort studies are susceptible to bias, particularly **recall bias** and **follow-up bias**, the tendency of some subjects to stop participating. **Confounding variables** can make it difficult to determine the variable truly associated with the outcome of interest.

For **retrospective cohort studies**, the existing records may lack the information sought. For **prospective cohort studies**, time and expense make them impractical in many cases. In the prospective cohort study example of adults involved in team sports, there must be funds for a dedicated staff to obtain and process the information over a period of 30–45 years. Turnover in study personnel will occur over the course of several decades, and methods for addressing these changes must be in place. Additional concerns include the loss of participants during follow-up and the inherent differences between those who remain in the study compared to those who do not (selection biases). Participants' recall of events since the previous survey may be faulty (recall bias) and some activities may be over- or under-reported (reporting bias). The results of the study may be influenced by other behaviors shared by the cohort that influence health outcomes after age 50, such as dietary habits, social engagement, and community environment (membership biases).

A further limitation of a longitudinal prospective cohort study is that publication will only be possible when data are evaluated at pre-selected intervals. For a new investigator trying to establish a publication record, working on other projects at the same time would be essential.

Hint: Do not get bogged down by the names of the study designs. If you find yourself confused between different study designs, start by answering the questions in Table 4.1. Once you have the information worked out, you can sort out what the study design is called.

Note: Additional guidance for designing an observational study involving retrospective chart reviews can be found in Chapter 7, Box 7.3.

EXPERIMENTAL STUDIES

The hallmark of any experimental study design, whether clinical or basic science, is that the investigator controls the intervention(s). Thus, experimental studies are also called **interventional studies**. Those who receive an **intervention** (the **experimental group**) are compared with those who do not (the **control group**). The control group may receive no intervention, a different intervention or a **placebo**—an intervention that has no therapeutic effect. Experimental studies are not limited to two groups; there may be multiple interventions worth testing.

For example, a study may include three experimental groups, each receiving a different dose of a medication and a control group receiving a placebo. Unlike observational studies, experimental designs can **identify cause-and-effect relationships**.

Between- and Within-Subjects Designs

Experimental designs come in two basic forms: **independent samples** (also called "between-subjects" designs) and **repeated measures** (also called "within-subjects" designs). The two formats reflect whether a single participant is assigned to only one group or to more than one group. In an independent samples experiment, the groups ("samples") are separate; there are different participants in every group. In contrast, with a repeated measures design, participants begin in one group then join another group. A participant may begin the study in the experimental group, and then switch to the control group, for example. Thus you "repeatedly measure" the same person under different conditions.

The study purpose usually determines whether independent samples or repeated measures are better suited to answering the research question. Depending on the research question, it may be beneficial to compare outcomes in the same participants. Does participant blood pressure decrease with a new medication (experimental) or daily meditation (control)? Advantages of a repeated measures design include the need for fewer participants and a greater likelihood of reaching statistical significance because the same participants are measured under both experimental and control conditions, thereby reducing between-subject variability (see Chapter 7 for further information on statistical significance).

When using repeated measures, the influence of initial group assignment must be considered. Ideally, each participant is randomly assigned to a first group. Thus, half of the participants are randomly selected to begin in the intervention group and half are randomly selected to begin in the control group. The impact of carry-over effects must also be considered. The effect of the intervention might linger into the control condition, or the control condition might impact the intervention. For example, the participants who practiced daily meditation may continue some habits after switching to the medication group. To ensure you address various concerns that might arise, it is helpful to work with a mentor or a statistician familiar with repeated measures to confirm whether your study design is optimal.

For many studies, it may be impossible, unethical, or undesirable to move subjects between groups. A participant in a study evaluating a surgical intervention could not switch to the control, non-surgical group, for example. In other cases, it may not be ethical or desirable to take a medication away from a patient, or it may not be possible to adequately address issues related to carry-over.

Randomization and Clinical Trials

Random assignment is a key feature of most experimental studies and is preferred for clinical research whenever possible and ethical. With randomization, every participant has an equal chance of being placed into any group. Random assignment presumably distributes the inherent differences between group members among the groups, thereby increasing the likelihood an observed effect is due to the intervention. Randomization does not eliminate all selection biases, however, and investigators need to carefully consider how they will identify and recruit participants (see also Chapter 5).

In some clinical studies, randomization may not be possible, desirable, or ethical. In such cases, non-randomized studies are completed. Participants do not have an equal chance of being placed in any group and may be assigned based on a clinical or demographic feature. Biases are more likely to occur without randomization and therefore investigators must consider where biases are likely to arise and develop ways to minimize them.

The **randomized control trial (RCT)** is considered the "**gold standard**" for medical research. When one thinks of RCT, large multicenter clinical trials designed to formally test new medications in humans may come to mind. These large clinical trials are usually conducted in four phases as described in **Box 4.2**. As a clinician you may have opportunities to assist with ongoing trials in your field if you are interested (**Box 4.3**).

RCTs also refer to studies of medical devices, surgical approaches, and gene therapies, as well as smaller studies, such as those conducted by a single investigator to compare two or more treatment approaches.

Clinical trials are generally set up using one of three common approaches: superiority, equivalence, or non-inferiority. Although similar in many respects, each approach is designed to answer a different question. Pharmaceutical studies are illustrated in the examples below, but the same approaches are used for non-pharmaceutical interventions.

> *Superiority trials* are designed to evaluate whether one treatment (the experimental treatment) is better than another (the control treatment). These are the most common form of clinical trial. Superiority trials are often used to test whether a new drug candidate is better than a placebo (control) or if a new drug or treatment is better than an existing one (control). Non-pharmaceutical interventions, such as exercise programs or behavioral modifications, can also be tested.

>***Equivalence trials*** are used to test if a new treatment (experimental group) is the same as an existing treatment (control group). To be considered the same, the results of the experimental group must fall within a predefined range, such as within 20% of the results from the control group. In pharmaceutical research, equivalence trials (also called bio-equivalence trials) are often used to show that the effect of a generic version of a drug is equal to the version already on the market.

>***Non-inferiority trials*** are conducted to test whether a new (experimental) treatment is no worse than the existing (control) treatment. The new treatment may be better than the control treatment, but the study is designed to only test whether the experimental treatment is no worse than the control treatment. Non-inferiority trials may be used to test whether a new medication is easier to administer, such as comparing a new oral medication to an existing injectable medication. Non-inferiority trials may also be used if using a placebo group is unethical. For example, in a clinical trial of a new chemotherapy medication, it would be unethical to give some patients a placebo instead of an existing, beneficial medication.

To limit potential biases, clinical trials usually involve at least one form of **blinding**. Blinding refers to concealing the treatment given to a participant. The participant, investigator, data analyst, or all three may be blinded to the treatment.

Examples:

1) A large, multicenter RCT evaluates a new drug for late-stage Parkinson's disease. The control group receives a placebo and neither the participants nor investigators know who receives which because the bottles and their contents look identical and are labeled with a code that is not deciphered until all data are collected. A placebo is allowed in this case because no existing standard of care is withheld. Investigators will have a data analyst unassociated with the study look at data at the midway point to see if there is evidence that the drug is providing benefits and, if so, may request to end the study early to allow others to benefit from the treatment. Conversely, the study also may be ended early if adverse effects are identified to limit further harm or risk to participants.

2) A faculty member at a single institution compares pain and functional outcomes over an 8-month period in patients who had surgery for carpal tunnel syndrome. One group receives standard of care using a traditional surgical approach, whereas the other has surgery with a newer modified approach that is accepted by the surgical community. Eligible participants are randomly assigned to receive one of the two surgical approaches but are not told which method they received. The surgeon does not select

which patients undergo which surgery and is informed of the group assignment on the day of surgery. An occupational therapist completes pain and functional assessments not knowing which surgery the patient received. All pre- and post-operative care is the same for both groups.

Ethical considerations and requirements: Experimental studies, including those that present minimal risk to participants, will require approval from the IRB. Investigators must document precisely what will happen to each participant and indicate if and how treatment differs from the standard of care. All risks and benefits to the participants will be explained, and methods for identifying and treating potential side effects will be detailed. If a placebo control is used, justification will be provided. Recruitment methods and informed consent procedures will be explained and the methods for reducing perceptions of coercion and undue influence will be detailed. All inclusion and exclusion criteria will be listed and justified. Any costs incurred by the participants will be explained. **CONSORT** (*Con*solidated *s*tandards *of r*eporting *t*rials) **guidelines**, listed at the end of this chapter, are followed for all clinical trials and most other experimental studies involving human subjects.

Statistical analysis: Experimental studies are evaluated with **inferential statistics**. Experimental studies are often framed to address null hypotheses such as: "The medication will not improve tremor in patients with Parkinson's disease," "There is no difference between group A and group B." **Descriptive statistics** may also be used to summarize additional data collected, such as that related to participant characteristics, and summary statistics of the groups.

Strengths: Experimental studies allow an investigator to **test one variable at a time** under controlled conditions, allowing for **replication** and potentially limiting confounding. Unlike observational studies, experimental studies can **indicate cause and effect**.

Limitations: Experimental studies tend to be **time consuming** and **expensive**. Only the interventions initiated at the beginning of the study can be evaluated. As with observational studies, investigators must consider **confounding variables** and identify methods that reduce them.

A further limitation of some experimental studies is that they create an **artificial situation** that limits generalizability. Further, **ethical concerns** regarding treatments given to experimental and control groups must be considered. As with all studies involving human subjects, the risks and benefits must be carefully considered, and any risks must be acceptable and fairly distributed among all participants.

For example, to evaluate a new drug, it may take several years to recruit and monitor the required number of patients. Funding will be needed to cover the costs of the medication and associated follow-up visits. The results may be difficult to interpret if the timing of medication relative to the stage of the disease was not optimal (timing bias), if the investigator unintentionally placed healthier patients in the treatment group (allocation bias), or if patients modified other behaviors because they were being observed (Hawthorne effect). Ethical concerns are likely to center around issues such as exposing participants to a treatment that could worsen symptoms or cause adverse effects, or depriving patients in the control group of a potentially beneficial new treatment.

Warning: Always review procedures and regulations regarding billing practices for patients enrolled in research studies. Failure to bill properly can lead to serious consequences for investigators and their institutions. Check if your institution has a committee or designated representative to evaluate what, if any, procedures can be billed to a participant's insurance company. If you do not know who to contact, check with your institution's IRB or sponsored programs and research office.

Box 4.2 Phases of Clinical Trials

There are four defined phases of clinical trials. The descriptions of the phases of clinical trials presented here use examples for testing a new drug candidate, but also apply to other interventions.

Phase I clinical trials are also called **safety trials**. These studies test the safety of the drug in a small group of healthy volunteers (usually about 20–100 participants) without a history or likelihood of having the condition the drug is intended to treat. Participants may be divided into groups that receive different doses of the drug. Outcome measures often include tolerance, absorption, distribution, metabolism, and excretion at a given dosage. Any adverse effects are reported. Phase I trials do not test the efficacy of the drug and do not include a comparison group.

If an existing drug with a known safety profile is being tested for another condition, investigators may receive approval to begin with phase II.

Phase II trials are the **initial clinical trials**. In this phase, safety is evaluated in participants with the condition the drug is intended to treat. Phase II includes a larger sample (usually about 100–400 participants) and a control group of patients who do not receive the drug. These trials are designed to evaluate the pharmacokinetics of the drug and adverse events in patients with the condition. However, efficacy is not evaluated in phase II trials.

Phase III or **full evaluation clinical trials** test the effectiveness of the treatment in a large group of participants (usually 500–3,000 or more) with the condition. These trials include a control group (with the condition) that does not receive the treatment. Participants are randomly assigned to the treatment or control group, unless there are clinical or ethical reasons not to use randomization. Phase III studies are designed to measure effectiveness of the drug for the condition it is intended to treat. Participants are monitored for improved outcomes as well as any adverse events. If the drug proves beneficial without risk of serious side effects, it may be approved for clinical use.

Phase IV trials, also called **post-market surveillance**, provide ongoing assessment of the safety of approved drugs. Phase IV tracks long-term effects and any serious adverse events that occur when using the drug. Phase IV trials may reveal benefits or risks that were not apparent during the phase III trials. Identified adverse events may lead to modifications of prescription recommendations or discontinuation of use.

Box 4.3   A Neuro-Hospitalist's Perspective: Becoming a Clinical Trial Investigator

Trevor Phinney, D.O.

Many of us who go into medicine want to make changes that improve the lives of our patients and enhance the future of medicine. Clinical trials are a direct way to help make such changes. At any given time, there are thousands of clinical trials happening throughout the world. These trials test various medical devices to improve surgical care, new and more efficient procedural pathways to enhance workflow and patient triage, and innovative medicines to alter current medical treatment for various disease processes. Becoming a part of groundbreaking medical studies takes a passion for your craft and the drive to want to make a difference.

Clinical trials are often sponsored by pharmaceutical companies or device manufacturers, who recruit physician co-investigators from various hospitals. Companies do not reach out to every hospital, however. They look for hospitals and investigators that serve the patient populations they are studying. To be an invited co-investigator you, or your institution, must have a track record of positive enrollment in previous trials. When a company sees that you recruit well and follow through on trials, you are likely to be invited to participate in upcoming trials.

If you want to be proactive, go to clinicaltrials.gov, a website with current clinical trials from over 200 countries. By searching keywords, you identify trials of interest to you. Reach out to the company to see if they are adding additional study sites. You will be asked about site feasibility, approximate number of patients you see annually for the pathology of interest, and an estimate of how many participants you could enroll at your site.

If you are enthusiastic about making a difference and changing the way medicine is practiced, clinical trials could be for you! By utilizing the above steps and maintaining your positive work ethic, you can become involved in numerous clinical trials to keep medicine moving forward.

4.3 CONCLUSIONS

Designing a new study is a creative stage of the research process in which you put your problem-solving skills to good use. You think about the question you want to answer, the information you would need to address that question, and how you could acquire that information. You begin with a general framework then refine your methods to develop a protocol suited to your question and resources.

Work closely with mentors, experienced investigators, and statisticians to make sure you design a study that will produce meaningful data. Follow the guidelines appropriate for your study approach (e.g., CARE, STROBE, CONSORT) to help organize your study and ensure you have considered all essential elements.

REFERENCES AND RESOURCES

BOOKS

Elmore JG, Wild D, Nelson HD, Katz DL. *Jekel's Epidemiology, Biostatistics, Preventive Medicine, and Public Health*. 5th ed. St. Louis: Elsevier; 2020.

Forister J, Blessing J. *Introduction to Research and Medical Literature for Health Professionals* 5th ed. Burlington: Jones & Bartlett Learning; 2020.

Jacobson K. *Introduction to Health Research Methods*. 3rd ed. Burlington: Jones & Bartlett Learning; 2021.

Hulley SB, Cummings SR, Browner WS, Grady DG, Newman TB. *Designing Clinical Research*. 4th ed. Philadelphia: Lippincott William & Wilkins: 2013.

ARTICLES

Andrade C. Understanding relative risk, odds ratio, and related terms: As simple as it can get. *J Clin Psychiatry*. 2015;76(7):e857–e861.

Andrade C. The primary outcome measure and its importance in clinical trials. *J Clin Psychiatry*. 2015;76(10):e1320–e1323.

Kapoor MC. Types of studies and research design. *Indian J Anaesth*. 2016;60(9):626–630.

Rezigalla AA. Observational study designs: Synopsis for selecting an appropriate study design. *Cureus*. 2020;12(1):e6692.

Vassar M, Holzmann M. The retrospective chart review: Important methodological considerations. *J Educ Eval Health Prof*. 2013;10:12.

Wang X, Kattan MW. Cohort studies: Design, analysis, and reporting. *Chest*. 2020;158(1S):S72–S78.

GUIDELINES FOR DIFFERENT STUDY DESIGNS

Checklists and guidelines are available to help investigators address important issues related to their study design. The following guidelines were developed for preparing a manuscript for a journal submission. Investigators will benefit from consulting these guidelines prior to beginning a study, before drafting a manuscript, and again before submission.

ARRIVE (for *A*nimal *r*esearch *r*eporting *in vivo* *e*xperiments)
- https://arriveguidelines.org/arrive-guidelines

CARE (for *C*ase *r*eports)
- www.care-statement.org

CONSORT (for *Con*solidated *s*tandards of *r*eporting *t*rials)
- www.consort-statement.org

PRISMA (for *P*referred *r*eporting *i*tems for *s*ystematic *r*eviews and *m*eta-*a*nalyses)
- www.prism-statement.org

SCARE (for *S*urgical *ca*se *r*eports)
- www.scareguideline.com

STROBE (for *St*rengthening the *r*eporting of *ob*servational studies in *e*pidemiology)
- www.strobe-statement.org

The Study Population: Finding and Enrolling Participants That Fit the Study Question

Lynne M. Bianchi, Ph.D. and Luke J. Rosielle, Ph.D.

Tips for Success:

Identify all characteristics of the desired target population.
Confirm your study population is representative of the target population.
Identify and address participant and investigator biases that could influence who completes the study.

Warning:

Failure to assemble a representative study population compromises the value of your data.

Key Concept: Appropriate and clearly defined procedures for assembling a study population increase the likelihood of obtaining meaningful results.

This chapter focuses on practices that help define and assemble an appropriate study population. Although specific methods for identifying and enrolling participants in a retrospective case-control study differ from those used to identify participants for a prospective randomized control trial, all strive to enroll those with the traits needed to answer the study question. **Because study outcomes reflect those who participate, your methods for assembling a representative population are critical to the success of the project**.

As you develop and revise your study plans, consider the **characteristics of the population appropriate to your research question**. Whether using an observational or experimental design, you must identify the desired target population and detail the criteria that make an individual eligible or ineligible for participation (**selection**). You decide how you will inform potential participants about the study (**recruitment**), how they will indicate their willingness to participate (**enrollment**), and how you will assign participants to different groups (**allocation**).

Note: Methods for unbiased recruitment and enrollment are introduced here and detailed further in Chapters 8 and 9.

DOI: 10.1201/9781003126478-5

Remember: If proper thought is not given to how you will recruit, select, enroll, and allocate your participants, you may end up with a **non-representative study population**, which means that your data will not accurately reflect the group you planned to study. In other words, your study will be flawed, and your data may be meaningless.

5.1 IDENTIFY WHO YOU WANT TO STUDY

During the earliest stages of study design, you define your **target population**, the group with the characteristics you wish to study. The target population may be large, such as all the males in the world, or smaller, such as all pregnant women between the ages of 25 and 35 years old in your city, or all adult patients with traumatic brain injury admitted to your hospital in the past 5 years. Whatever the size, you are unlikely to study every person in the target population. Therefore, you will define methods to select a subset of that target population. You will define **inclusion criteria**, the characteristics that make potential participants eligible to be in the study, and **exclusion criteria**, those characteristics that make individuals ineligible to participate.

Common inclusion or exclusion criteria are age, gender, and disease status. Other considerations are the ability to complete the study tasks and willingness to report for follow-up visits. To ensure generalizability, studies should include as many representative individuals as possible. Therefore, list as few exclusion criteria as feasible, given your study purpose. Some exclusion criteria are usually necessary, however. You cannot study adolescent sleep patterns in 30- to 40-year-old adults, and you cannot study pregnancy in males. However, you do not exclude a group of individuals based on convenience or arbitrary criteria. **Except for valid scientific or ethical reasons, studies should include men, women and children**.

You will, however, need to balance broad inclusion with the need to reduce confounding variables. For example, you may exclude individuals who had specific illnesses or surgeries because those could interfere with interpretation of treatment outcomes, or you may need to exclude those who are not fluent in English if they would have difficulty understanding and answering questions on a survey.

The **source** or **accessible population** includes all eligible members of the target population that you can contact. These may be individuals in your geographic area or healthcare system, members of a professional or patient society, or those listed in a database (**Box 5.1**).

Members of the source population who are invited to participate in the study form the **sample population**. Those who choose to enroll in your study become the **study population**, the group from which you will analyze your findings. Because all your data will come from this group of individuals, it is **critical to assemble a study population that represents the target population**.

Note: Define inclusion and exclusion criteria for every study. Investigators usually know to consider inclusion and exclusion criteria for prospective studies but sometimes overlook their importance in retrospective designs, such as chart reviews.

Tip: **When defining inclusion or exclusion criteria, be sure you have accurate methods to confirm eligibility.** For example, how would you confirm pregnancy status, ability to follow directions, drug abuse history, length of medication use, or current dementia status? Too often, investigators list the criteria before realizing they cannot confirm participant status in one or more areas. It is also important to identify who has the necessary expertise to determine eligibility status. Is anyone on your study team qualified to diagnose dementia? If necessary, you may need to include additional study personnel.

Remember: Clearly defined inclusion and exclusion criteria must be applied accurately by all team members during recruitment and enrollment phases of the study to ensure the desired study population is assembled.

5.2 DEFINE THE SAMPLING METHOD

For some studies, every eligible member of your source population may be invited to participate. This is usually possible when the source population is relatively small and easy to identify; for example, all second-year residents at your institution. However, for other studies, your source population will be too large. In those instances, sampling strategies can help you identify representative participants from the larger source population.

Sampling methods are divided into two primary categories: probability sampling and non-probability sampling. **Probability sampling methods** are designed so that **every individual in the source population has an equal chance** of being selected to participate. Examples include notifying all college students in the United States, all patients with breast cancer in Minnesota, all adult patients in a hospital.

Non-probability sampling methods do not give everyone in the source population an equal chance of being selected. Inviting college students from a single course at a local university or patients from one clinic does not include everyone from the source population; it only includes a subset you presume represents the larger population.

USE PROBABILITY SAMPLING METHODS FOR MOST EXPERIMENTAL STUDIES

Probability sampling methods are typically used in **experimental studies** and most often **involve random selection**, the chance selection of a given participant. The **time and expense** associated with probability sampling is often greater than with non-probability methods. Yet, whenever study design and resources allow, probability sampling methods should be used as they help **reduce sampling bias** and **improve generalizability**.

> ***Simple random sampling*** means every individual in the population has an equal chance of being selected for the study. For example, a

random sample of all the patients with breast cancer listed in a national database is selected using a random number generator. **Random number generators** provide lists of numbers to indicate who in the population will be contacted. Computerized or printed versions of random number generators are available. For example, if you want to study 400 people and have an alphabetical list of 1500 patients, you would first number each name from 1 through 1500. The random number generator would then identify 400 numbers, and the patients with the corresponding number would be contacted. Because each name on the list has an equal chance of being selected, randomization is achieved.

Systematic random sampling means a subset of the population is selected using a consistent method. For example, a sample of all patients in a database is identified by selecting every twenty-fifth name on the list.

Stratified random sampling involves dividing potential participants into strata (subgroups) based on characteristics, particularly potential confounding variables. For example, drinkers and non-drinkers are stratified into two groups; runners, walkers, and wheelchair athletes are stratified into three groups. A predetermined number of individuals from each stratum is then randomly selected.

Cluster sampling divides all members of a large target population, such as a geographic region, into subgroups (clusters). Each cluster is assigned a number. The sample may include all individuals in randomly selected clusters or a randomly selected subpopulation within those randomly selected clusters. For example, a city or county is divided into 16 areas (clusters) from which 5 are chosen at random. All households in the 5 clusters are sent a survey. Alternatively, 750 households in each of the 5 clusters are randomly selected to receive the survey.

CONSIDER COMMON NON-PROBABILITY SAMPLING METHODS IF APPROPRIATE

Non-probability methods are typically used in **observational studies** and some experimental studies. Non-probability sampling methods are generally **easier, faster**, and **less expensive** than the probability sampling methods and are therefore also used for **pilot studies**. However, because non-probability sampling methods do not give everyone in the source population an equal chance of being selected, these methods are subject to more **biases** and **limited generalizability**.

Convenience sampling means any eligible individual who is readily **available to the investigator** is invited to join the study. These are individuals who are easily identified and contacted, such as patients treated at a single clinic or students in an introductory biology course at a local university.

The ease of contact makes this **one of the most common forms of non-probability sampling**. However, patients who attend your clinic may differ in some ways from people who attend another clinic in your city, or a clinic in another region of the country. College students who take introductory biology may be different from students who do not take that class and students who take the course at one university may differ from those at another. Thus, study populations obtained by convenience sampling may not fully represent the target population.

> *Consecutive sampling* is a **subtype of convenience sampling** that enrolls groups of participants over a longer period. For example, individuals may be chosen at three different times during a year.

The goal of consecutive sampling is **to reduce potential differences in members of the source population that arise at different times**. Patients who live in a cold climate and come to a clinic in the winter, for example, likely differ in some ways from those who do not. Those who do not come in the winter may have mobility issues or may be living in a different area of the country during colder months. Students who enroll in summer sections of a course may be motivated to work ahead or may be behind in course credits and trying to catch up. In every example, if selection only occurred at a single time in the year, the resulting study population would differ in some ways from the rest of the source population.

> *Snowball sampling* refers to a method in which **participants identify others** who may meet enrollment criteria.

Although this approach limits how well the sample represents the target population, it may be beneficial if the **target population is small** or **difficult to identify**. For example, participants may identify other mothers who use non-pasteurized milk, a practice that tends to be uncommon and may not be openly shared.

> *Purposive or judgmental sampling* is based on **investigator knowledge**. For example, an investigator may identify which clinical site is best for recruiting participants based on knowledge of patient demographics. Another investigator may invite patients based on knowledge of patients' occupational history.

Note: Whenever participants identify other potential participants (snowballing), or investigators select participants based on their knowledge of a population (purposive), there will likely be more similarities among members of the identified population than would be found in the target population.

Tip: Non-probability sampling is common in many resident-initiated research projects. Always **consider how your sample may differ from the target population and how those differences are likely to influence your results**. Be sure to include such limitations in the discussion section of your publications and presentations.

Hint: To help **decrease the inherent biases** that arise from non-probability sampling, participants should be **randomly assigned** to groups whenever possible.

Box 5.1   Finding Participants in Databases

There are many local and national databases that compile information on patients with certain conditions or treatment histories, such as those with heart disease or those who have received anesthesia. You may be able to access these for your studies. For example, you may be given access to de-identified information, or you might request permission to contact individuals who consented to release their contact information for research purposes. Your inclusion and exclusion criteria would then be applied to the subjects in the database or datasets.

Tip: The **National Health and Nutrition Examination Survey** maintained by the United States Centers for Disease Control and Prevention can be used to answer some research questions.

5.3 LIMIT BIASES THAT INTERFERE WITH ASSEMBLING A REPRESENTATIVE POPULATION

Whenever a study population does not reflect the same diversity as the target population, generalizability is limited. To include participants who represent the target population, you must eliminate or reduce practices that discourage or omit eligible participants. **Biases,** also called systematic errors, can occur at every stage of the process. For example, **selection bias** occurs when the inclusion or exclusion criteria are too strict. **Recruitment bias** is a concern if the study is only advertised at a single clinic or a few similar clinics. **Enrollment bias** is a problem when an investigator describes the study in such a way that encourages or discourages some individuals to participate. **Allocation bias** occurs when an investigator assigns participants with certain characteristics to one group and those with other characteristics to another.

Participant and investigator biases are among the most common biases you will confront when assembling your study population. Most biases are unintentional and difficult to recognize. Although biases are part of every study, you can eliminate or reduce many of them by thoroughly reviewing your selection, recruitment, enrollment, and allocation strategies.

PARTICIPANT BIASES IMPACT WHO JOINS AND COMPLETES A STUDY

Volunteer and non-responder biases are the two primary forms of participant bias that nearly every study must consider. **Volunteer bias** reflects the fact that individuals who choose to participate in a study are different in some ways from those who do not volunteer. Similarly, those who do not participate (**non-responders**) are different in some ways from those who do. Non-response bias includes those who decline to participate, those who are difficult to reach, and those who fail to follow-up once enrolled in a study.

To increase participation of those less likely to volunteer, investigators should consider multiple methods of contact including phone, email, direct mail, and in-person communication. For some populations, snowball sampling may be useful.

> *Attrition bias* is the loss of study participants during the follow-up period. The inherent differences between those who continue and those who do not will likely impact the study results in some way. For example, there will be some differences in those who are able to and choose to follow-up, those who are able but choose *not* to follow-up, and those who are unable to follow-up. Depending on your study, these differences could skew your data in various ways. For example, people for whom a treatment is not working may drop out of a study. The data may then suggest the treatment is more effective because most of the data come from those who received benefit.

In all cases, it is important to identify and implement ways to minimize attrition. The number, duration, and location of follow-up visits should be considered when planning your study, and methods for encouraging and assisting with follow-up should be developed.

> *Recall bias* occurs when a potential participant does not accurately recall information. In some cases, a person may have forgotten details of health information or may recall events inaccurately.

Recall bias can impact the accuracy of eligibility as well as that of the data collected. Whenever possible, methods to confirm reported information should be used. For example, you might ask questions in different ways to see if the same response is given or review medical records of enrolled participants to confirm information.

INVESTIGATOR BIASES INFLUENCE HOW PARTICIPANTS ARE IDENTIFIED AND ASSIGNED TO GROUPS

> *Selection and recruitment bias* result whenever **eligible members are excluded, or appear to be excluded,** from the study. For example, if the target population includes all adult contact lens wearers aged 18–32 years, but the study is only announced on a college campus, where most students are under the age of 25, the study population will not be inclusive of all ages under investigation. If the study only enrolls those treated at a clinic specializing in eye diseases, those enrolled will differ in some ways from contact lens wearers who do not have need of a specialty clinic. If inclusion criteria state male or female, those who are non-binary may feel they are ineligible to participate.

To limit such biases, investigators should define inclusion and exclusion criteria as broadly as possible, and review materials for any content that could misrepresent eligibility or discourage participation. Recruitment should occur in multiple formats and at as many sites as feasible.

> *Enrollment bias* occurs whenever an investigator or other **study team member influences who joins the study**. It is essential to have clearly defined methods for identifying, screening, and enrolling participants. It is equally important to monitor that the approved methods are used consistently. For example, some who enroll participants may tend to highlight the positive aspects of the study but downplay potential risks. Others, as they try to present the study in a neutral manner, may inadvertently discourage participation. Some may present the study in a positive manner to those they identify as "good candidates" and in a less favorable manner to those they deem "poor candidates."

To limit such biases, methods for screening candidates and identifying eligible participants should be reviewed with all members of the study team. Rehearsing enrollment scenarios can further improve consistency among team members.

Assessing characteristics of participants enrolled by different investigators early in the process may identify areas to be addressed. For example, if a study is designed to assess the effects of a diet plan on individuals with chronic obstructive pulmonary disease (COPD) of any severity (stage 1–4) but one of the team members enrolling patients does not think those with a mild form of COPD (stage 1) are sick, the study population would be skewed to participants with moderate or severe cases. However, if enrollment characteristics were reviewed after the first 2 weeks, the biased enrollment could be identified and corrected.

> *Allocation bias* is a concern when participants are not randomly assigned to a group. For example, an investigator may assign those who appear healthier to the control group leading to skewed baseline data. To prevent participant characteristics from influencing group assignment, it is beneficial to have participants randomly allocated. **Random assignment (allocation)** gives each participant an equal chance of being in any group.

A further means of limiting allocation bias is through allocation concealment. **Allocation concealment** means the person enrolling participants does not know to which group any individual will be assigned. Sealed envelopes might be used to determine which group a participant joins. The assignment remains unknown until the envelope is opened. This is a form of **blinding**.

It is also best if those involved with the study are not aware of their group assignment, that is, participants are **blinded** to the treatment.

Blinding may refer to the investigator, participant, or individuals doing the data analysis. Studies have traditionally been reported to be single, double, or triple blinded. A single-blinded study typically referred to participants being unaware of which treatment they received, whereas a double-blinded study usually meant that both participant and investigator were unaware of the treatment given. A triple-blinded study would signify that the participants, investigators, and data analysts were all unaware of which treatment was given to any individual.

Due to the ambiguity of who is blinded to what, particularly in a single- or double-blinded study, those terms are now discouraged. Instead of saying the study was single-blinded, you should state that participants were blinded to their group assignment. Instead of saying you conducted a double-blinded study, state that participants and investigators were blinded to group assignment.

Tip: If random selection is not possible or desirable, random allocation should be used.

Note: Randomization and blinding are often used in experimental studies but may not be feasible in observational studies. For example, in a case-control or cohort study design, where the exposure (risk factor) or outcome (disease) is known, random assignment and blinding are not possible.

Remember: **Participation in a study is voluntary** and study team members must never try to persuade or coerce participation. Review all ethical practices and approved consent documents with team members before contacting any potential participants (see Chapters 8 and 9).

5.4 CONCLUSIONS

Assembling a study population suitable for answering your research question is an essential part of the study design process. Defining inclusion and exclusion criteria, and applying appropriate sampling, recruitment, enrollment, and allocation methods to limit bias are crucial steps. The success of every project depends on thoughtful planning and ongoing review of procedures to ensure the study sample represents the intended target population. Whenever necessary, collaborate with others to ensure you are effectively reaching all members of the target population.

REFERENCES AND RESOURCES

BOOKS

Jacobson K. *Introduction to Health Research Methods*. 3rd ed. Burlington: Jones & Bartlett Learning; 2021.

Hulley SB, Cummings SR, Browner WS, Grady DG, Newman TB. *Designing Clinical Research*. 4th ed. Philadelphia: Lippincott William & Wilkins; 2013.

ARTICLES

Elfil M, Negida A. Sampling methods in clinical research; an educational review. *Emerg (Tehran)*. 2017;5(1):e52.

Martínez-Mesa J, González-Chica DA, Duquia RP, et al. Sampling: How to select participants in my research study? *An Bras Dermatol*. 2016;91(3):326–330.

Valerio MA, Rodriguez N, Winkler P, et al. Comparing two sampling methods to engage hard-to-reach communities in research priority setting. *BMC Med Res Methodol*. 2016;16(1):146.

Wallington SF, Dash C, Sheppard VB, et al. Enrolling minority and underserved populations in cancer clinical research. *Am J Prev Med*. 2016;50(1):111–117.

Wieland ML, Njeru JW, Alahdab F, et al. Community-engaged approaches for minority recruitment into clinical research: A scoping review of the literature. *Mayo Clin Proc*. 2021;96(3):733–743.

CHAPTER 6

Collecting Data You Can Trust

Lynne M. Bianchi, Ph.D. and Luke J. Rosielle, Ph.D.

Tips for Success:

> Choose methods that collect valid and reliable data.
> Identify likely sources of errors and develop ways to minimize them.
> Confirm everyone on the study team uses data collection methods
>   correctly.

Warning:

> Procedures for correcting mistakes must be ethical, consistent, and
>   clearly documented.

Key Concept: Errors and mistakes are part of every study. Careful attention to data collection procedures limits the impact of these on study outcomes.

Part of the research design process includes selecting which instruments will be used to collect the information you seek. A study may collect data from questionnaires/surveys, rating scales, laboratory tests, medical images, clinical records, or some combination of sources. Whatever the planned methods, the instruments must measure what they are intended to measure. The instruments must also be properly used. You will need to be certain everyone on the study team follows the specified protocols for collecting and recording data. Without proper attention to these aspects of the study, you risk collecting data that does not answer the study question.

This chapter outlines practices to help you and your team members collect and record trustworthy data.

6.1 REDUCE SYSTEMATIC AND RANDOM ERRORS: CHOOSE VALID AND RELIABLE DATA COLLECTION METHODS

As an investigator, your goal is to collect data that represent the true values of the variables studied. How well your data represent the true values will be influenced by the validity and reliability of your materials and methods.

Valid measures are **accurate**; they always **measure what they are were intended to measure**. Examples include a blood test for syphilis that identifies syphilis, and survey questions that are correctly interpreted by participants.

DOI: 10.1201/9781003126478-6

Reliable measures are **precise**; they produce the **same measurement each time**. For example, a scale measures 45 kilograms every time 45 kilograms is placed on the scale, and an answer to a survey question is the same each time a participant is asked.

Unfortunately, data collection is always susceptible to errors. **An error is anything that misrepresents the true value**. Errors may be due to issues with an instrument, investigator, or participant. Errors may be **systematic**, meaning they are consistent, or **random**, meaning that they occur by chance.

When choosing instruments and defining procedures, look for potential sources of errors and develop ways to reduce or eliminate their impact on your data collection.

VALID MEASUREMENTS LACK SYSTEMATIC ERRORS

Systematic errors, or **biases**, cause consistent changes in a measurement. Although the changes are consistent, the values are always inaccurate. For example, an instrument which consistently leads to the underdiagnosis of a disease in one ethnic or age group, but not others, is a systematically biased instrument. **Valid measurements**, in contrast, are accurate and **lack systematic error**.

Statistics cannot correct for systematic errors. Therefore, it is important to confirm the validity of your measurement tools and monitor how team members use them.

There are several potential sources of biases to consider.

Instrument bias results from inaccuracies in the instrument or the method of data collection. For example, a thermometer may consistently read two degrees lower than the actual temperature. A question may be worded in such a way that it prompts a particular response. The question, "You do not drink alcohol, do you?" is more likely to receive the answer of "no" than the question "Do you drink alcohol?"

To reduce instrument bias, **calibrate equipment** before each use, **use a second instrument** to confirm results, review the wording of questions, and **ask multiple questions** designed to elicit the same response.

Investigator (observer) bias occurs whenever a team member makes the same measurement error repeatedly. Like other biases, this usually arises without the investigator realizing a change in behavior. For example, an investigator may unknowingly ask a question one way to female participants but a different way to male participants. Another might round up body weight for patients perceived as underweight but not for those who appear obese.

To reduce investigator bias, **develop standard protocols**, **review them with team members**, and **monitor performance** throughout the study.

Participant bias occurs when inaccurate information is provided by someone enrolled in the study. For example, answers to survey questions may vary depending on who asks the questions. On a rating scale, the answers may reflect a participant's preferred way of answering. Some participants may always select the lowest options, and others may always choose the middle options.

To limit the effects of such biases, **ask for information in multiple ways**. In some cases, patterns may emerge that confirm participant bias. For example, participants who always select the lowest rating on a scale will choose the lowest ratings for both "My doctor encourages me to discuss my health concerns" and "I do not think my doctor wants me to share concerns about my health."

Note: If you are trying to assess a construct that is in any way complex or multifaceted ("depression," for example), it is usually best to **use an established, peer-reviewed valid instrument** rather than develop your own. Choose instruments that have gone through a rigorous construction process, have well-established psychometric properties, and have been extensively tested.

Tip: If a judgment about a subjective quality of the participant is needed (e.g., how well or unwell a patient appears), multiple raters can assess each participant. The principal investigator will monitor the responses of the various raters and retrain study team members or revise methods if there is too much inter-rater variability in the responses.

Hint: Whenever possible, use surveys/questionnaires previously shown to be valid. Check how validity was determined and remember that publication in a journal does not confirm validity.

Remember: Review all measurement tools and practice administering tests before working with participants.

RANDOM ERRORS CREATE VARIABILITY

Random errors cause **unpredictable measurements**. Some measurements will be higher than the true value whereas others will be lower. How different any given measure is from the true value is unknown and variable. Random errors are not systematic; they do not affect one outcome more than any other. Thus, random errors produce **variability**.

Statistical methods account for variability. When an error is random and the sample size is large enough, an estimate of the true value can be calculated. However, it is still important to identify sources of variability and limit their impact on data collection. Like systematic errors, random errors can be attributed to instruments, investigators, or participants, and, though unpredictable, their impact can be reduced by establishing standardized procedures.

>*Instrument variability* occurs when a measurement tool fluctuates in unknown ways. The accuracy of a laboratory scale may change throughout the day based in part on the temperature and humidity in the room. A survey question may be perceived differently by different participants; the question, "How much do you drink daily?" may be interpreted by some to mean all liquids consumed and by others to refer to alcohol consumption.

Instrument variability can be limited by establishing **standard procedures**, including the time and location of measurements. Ambiguous survey questions can be identified by others outside the research team and corrected prior to administration. A pilot study with members of the target population may be beneficial.

>*Investigator variability* occurs when inconsistent measurements are made by a member of the research team. For example, an investigator may ask questions differently or eliminate some questions based on an experience with a previous participant. An investigator may read the volume in a syringe from different angles each time, causing some volumes to be higher and others lower than the intended amount.

Investigators should **practice** using equipment, taking measurements, and administering surveys prior to working with participants.

Standard procedures and repeated measures can also help control for **intra-rater variability** that occurs when one investigator obtains a different measurement each time and **inter-rater variability** that occurs when different measurements are obtained by different investigators.

The number of team members taking measurements should be limited to those necessary as **the more people involved, the more opportunities exist for investigator error**.

>*Participant variability* arises from inherent biological and behavioral differences that cannot be anticipated or controlled. Examples include an individual's unpredictable differences in blood pressure readings throughout the day, and differences in participants who complete a cognitive assessment without difficulty after an 8-hour fast, and those who are unable to focus after a few hours without food.

Although it is not possible to eliminate such variability, following **standardized procedures** and taking **measurements** in the same manner and setting each time will reduce additional sources of variability. For example, if a study requires weekly blood pressure measurements, checking blood pressure 5 minutes after a participant is settled in a comfortable chair eliminates variability that would arise if the participant's blood pressure were measured on an office examination table some weeks and in a comfortable chair other weeks. Standardized procedures would also reduce variability between participants whose blood pressure is taken in one setting *versus* another. Biological variability would not be addressed, only confounding variables associated with the setting.

Like investigator variability, the impact of participant variability can be reduced by **repeating measurements**.

Note: A tool may be reliable, but the person using it may not be. Proper training and monitoring help ensure measurements are taken reliably each time by all investigators.

Remember: Investigators are responsible for evaluating the instruments used to collect data. You must confirm that each tool used is **valid** (accurate) and **reliable** (precise). Any clinical tests used must be **sensitive** and **specific** (Box 6.1)

Box 6.1   Sensitive and Specific Tests

If your study includes clinical tests, you need to consider their sensitivity and specificity.

Sensitivity is the **probability** that the results will be **positive** in **patients with the disease or condition** you are evaluating.

Sensitive tests are good for **screening** since they are unlikely to miss someone with the disease. They are used to rule out a disease or condition because a person is unlikely to have the disease when a sensitive test is negative.

Specificity is the **probability** that the results will be **negative** in patients **without the disease**.

Specific tests are good for **confirming** a diagnosis. Because the test will be negative for those without that disease or condition, a positive result from a specific test supports a diagnosis.

6.2 DESIGN EASY-TO-USE DATA COLLECTION SHEETS

In research, errors, whether systematic or random, are different from mistakes. A mistake occurs when an investigator accidentally writes down the wrong number on a data collection sheet or places test results in the wrong folder. Mistakes are likely to occur in any study, and, while you cannot prevent them all, you can develop practices to minimize them.

One way to limit mistakes is to think about the information you will record and how you will record it. You use a **data collection sheet** or **data collection tool** to record the data. For many studies, the data collection tool is a spreadsheet that is also used for statistical analysis. How you design your data collection tool will influence how easy it is to record and analyze your data.

Your data likely will be gathered from multiple sources. Some information may come from patient medical records, some from tests you administer, and some from participant surveys or rating scales. Therefore, **time spent developing an easy-to-follow data collection tool is time well spent**. For example, if your study requires information from patient charts, think about where that information is organized in the medical record. To improve the ease and speed of data collection, organize your data collection tool to match the organization of the medical record. If participant gender and age appear on the first page of the medical record, this information should be listed among the first columns of the data collection tool. Thus, **rather than organizing your columns based on your primary interests, put them in an order that makes data entry easiest**.

If your study includes **categorical data**, decide how that will be recorded in the spreadsheet. Numerical values can be assigned to each categorical variable to aid subsequent data analysis. For example, "left-handed" may be entered as 1 and "right-handed" entered as 2. Make sure everyone who enters the data understands the system you develop. Alternatively, enter words or abbreviations, then have one person go through the final data set to convert everything to numerical values. The find/replace function in most spreadsheets can easily recode words into numbers. Keep the original file to compare for accuracy.

If multiple people are entering data, make sure each person enters the data using consistent nomenclature. If words are used, it is important that they are always entered in the same format, including spelling and capitalization. Some statistical packages will treat "male," "Male", and "M" as three separate categories, so consistency is essential.

Though numbers may be easier to enter than words, a key is required to interpret what the numbers represent. Due to the arbitrary nature of the numbers associated with nominal variables, it does not make sense to perform any arithmetic on these results. Computing the "average gender" does not give meaningful information. However, nominal variables can be counted for statistical analysis of the frequency at which something occurred. Thus, those who analyze the data must be informed of what the numbers represent to ensure that the correct analyses are done.

Also note that, for **statistical purposes, interval** (no true 0 values exist) **and ratio variables** (true 0 values exist) **are generally treated as equivalent**. Thus, the same kinds of statistics are used for interval variables and ratio variables. The practical difference involves their interpretation. Because ratios always reflect consistent, measurable differences, you can make multiplicative statements. For example, 10 seconds is twice as fast as 5 seconds, and 100 kilograms is twice as heavy as 50 kilograms. In contrast, no such claim can be made for interval variables; 100° Fahrenheit is not twice as warm as 50° Fahrenheit.

Always record your data with the highest level of measurement possible. As noted in Chapter 4, there are benefits to recording available ratio or interval data rather than recording that information as categorical or ordinal data. You can later convert patient age or weight to a categorical or ordinal ranking, but you cannot convert a set of categories or rankings to an exact age or weight.

For example, researchers often divide participant ages into arbitrary groups such as: 0–5 years, 6–10 years, 11–15 years, 16–20 years, and 21+ years. However, doing so takes a variable that is naturally a ratio (age) and records it as an ordinal variable. Not only is information lost, but the investigator is now restricted in the types of statistics that can be done with the data.

A second problem with grouping ratios such as ages is that they are usually arbitrary. Are the experiences of those aged 0–5 sufficiently similar that they warrant being grouped together? Is a 22-year-old more like a 56-year-old or an 18-year-old? If you ever choose to divide a continuous variable, be sure there is a strong, empirical justification for how data are grouped.

If your study includes participant age, it is best to record the date of birth or age at the time of the study and later convert participant ages to groups, if helpful.

Tip: Review your data collection document on a regular basis. Identify mistakes before it is too late to correct them.

Note: If you receive grant funding, the sponsoring agency may require that you collect certain types of information from participants, such as age, gender, and ethnicity. Decide how you will use this information before you begin data collection. For example, you may choose to report some data to the agency using descriptive statistics or to analyze and publish the data using inferential statistics.

6.3 FORMALIZE PROCEDURES FOR DEALING WITH MISTAKES

Mistakes are made during every study. Some mistakes are obvious and can be easily corrected, whereas others cannot. When reviewing data, it may be obvious that an adult participant was not born 10 years ago. You may have other records that indicate the correct date of birth, or you may be able to ask the participant directly. However, if you noticed the error after participant information was de-identified you would not be able to correct the mistake.

Because mistakes are likely, investigators should be prepared to deal with them when they occur. For example, if a participant's blood pressure is remarkably different on one occasion, you may suspect someone switched that participant's data with another participant's. However, you cannot simply change presumptive errors without confirmation. In some cases, you may have to eliminate a single data point from analysis whereas at other times you will have to exclude all the data collected for that participant.

What will your study team do when mistakes are detected or suspected? **Before you begin a study, establish protocols for dealing with mistakes**. Try to envision as many mistakes as you can, however unlikely they may seem. **The process of identifying potential sources of mistakes often prevents them from occurring in the first place**.

Any mistakes must be dealt with in an **ethical and consistent manner**. You should determine who will be responsible for correcting mistakes and how the mistakes and any corrections will be documented. If you need to eliminate data due to mistakes, report how much data were eliminated in any subsequent presentations or publications.

6.4 CONCLUSIONS

Systematic errors, random errors, and mistakes are issues that must be addressed in every study. To collect data you can trust, you must spend time choosing and refining study protocols and data collection procedures. It is important to identify potential sources of errors and implement procedures to reduce their likelihood of occurring. Be sure to create clearly defined protocols and review them regularly with all team members. Design a data collection tool that is easy to follow and establish methods for correcting and documenting mistakes.

REFERENCES AND RESOURCES

BOOKS

Elmore JG, Wild D, Nelson HD, Katz DL. *Jekel's Epidemiology, Biostatistics, Preventive Medicine, and Public Health*. 5th ed. St. Louis: Elsevier; 2020.

Hulley SB, Cummings SR, Browner WS, Grady DG, Newman TB. *Designing Clinical Research*. 4th ed. Philadelphia:Lippincott William & Wilkins; 2013.

Tamim H. *Introduction to Clinical Research for Residents*. Riyadh: Saudi Commission for Health Specialties; 2014.

Testa MA, Simonson DC. The use of questionnaires and surveys. In: Robertson D and Williams GH eds. *Clinical and Translational Science*. 2nd ed. London: Elsevier; 2017.

ARTICLES

Rickards G, Magee C, Artino AR Jr. You can't fix by analysis what you've spoiled by design: Developing survey instruments and collecting validity evidence. *J Grad Med Educ*. 2012;4(4):407–410.

Trevethan R. Sensitivity, specificity, and predictive values: Foundations, liabilities, and pitfalls in research and practice. *Front Public Health*. 2017;5:307.

CHAPTER 7

Preparing Studies for Statistical Analysis

Luke J. Rosielle, Ph.D. and Lynne M. Bianchi, Ph.D.

Tips for Success:

> If you require assistance with statistics, or think you may, consult with a statistician early in the process.
>
> Before beginning any study, confirm you are collecting the data needed for statistical analysis.

Warning:

> Statistics only evaluate the question(s) addressed in your study. They do not "find" statistically significant differences for you.

Key Concept: The research question, study design, variables, distribution, and number of groups determine the statistical tests to use.

Once collected, your data will be analyzed using various statistical tests to help you interpret the findings. This chapter explains how to frame a hypothesis for statistical analysis, calculate an appropriate sample size, and differentiate characteristics of frequently used statistical methods.

The importance of setting up your study properly from the beginning cannot be overemphasized. Far too many studies are completed with insufficient or incorrect data, leaving investigators with no meaningful results to share. If you are unfamiliar with the terms presented in this chapter, have limited experience with statistical analysis, or need to evaluate larger data sets with more advanced techniques, make sure you consult with an experienced mentor or statistician. Advice on what to prepare prior to meeting with a statistician is provided in Box 7.1.

Note: Some of the terms in this chapter were introduced in Chapter 4 and are included in Appendix A.

Tip: Review the study design examples in Chapter 4 to see which statistical tests are appropriate for your chosen study designs.

7.1 KNOW WHEN AND HOW TO FRAME RESEARCH QUESTIONS FOR HYPOTHESIS TESTING

Statistical methods are divided into two broad categories: descriptive statistics and inferential statistics. **Descriptive statistics** provide information on the

DOI: 10.1201/9781003126478-7

measures of **central tendency** (e.g., mean, median) and the **variability** (the spread) of the data (e.g., standard deviation, range). They **cannot be used to test hypotheses**. Descriptive statistics are used to evaluate data collected in **observational studies** and may summarize some data from experimental studies.

In contrast, **inferential statistics** are **used to formally test a hypothesis**. These methods calculate values (e.g., *p*-values and **confidence intervals**) to indicate the likelihood the data reflect true differences among groups. **Analytical observational** and **experimental studies** phrase research questions in terms of a hypothesis.

DEFINE NULL AND ALTERNATIVE HYPOTHESES FOR INFERENTIAL STATISTICS

Hypotheses are framed to test the **null hypothesis**, the hypothesis that an intervention/exposure does *not* make a difference. This ends up being an important conceptual point—statistical tests operate only on the null hypothesis, and the results of the statistical test will tell you, given your data, the likelihood that your null hypothesis (or "null") is true (there is likely no difference among groups). If the probability that the null is true ends up being very small (a probability called the "*p*-value"), then the most reasonable conclusion is that the null is false (there likely is a difference among groups). The **alternative hypothesis**, that the intervention makes a difference, is **accepted by default if the null hypothesis is rejected**. Note, however, that **the alternative hypothesis cannot be directly tested**, even though that is usually the hypothesis of interest to the investigator.

If you want to know if an intervention helps patients, you test the null hypothesis to determine the likelihood that there is no difference among the groups. **If the likelihood of the null being correct is very small, you have found statistical significance**, and therefore accept the alternative hypothesis. The logic may appear to be a little backwards for newcomers to statistics, but this is what is meant by "statistical significance." For example, imagine you are interested in whether an occupational therapy treatment protocol (intervention/exposure) will reduce the amount of pain medication (outcome) taken by patients aged 65–95 with osteoarthritis of the thumb. Your *null hypothesis* is that patients receiving occupational therapy will be indistinguishable from patients who do not receive occupational therapy in terms of the amount of pain medication taken; in other words, occupational therapy does not change how much pain medication is used by a participant.

When you conduct the appropriate statistical test, the resulting *p*-value tells you the probability that the null hypothesis is true (no difference between the two groups). You likely developed the study because you suspected that occupational therapy will be effective, so you anticipate that the null will be false, and the *p*-value will be very small, for example 0.05 or less. However, if statistical analysis indicates there is no difference between those who receive occupational therapy and those who do not (p is greater than 0.05, or 5%), the null hypothesis is accepted. **You cannot prove that the null is true; the best you can say is that you have insufficient evidence to reject the null**.

If the results of the statistical test tell you there is less than a 5% chance the null is true ($p < 0.05$), you have found statistical significance and the null hypothesis is rejected. In this example, if there is a statistically significant decrease in the amount of pain medication taken by those receiving occupational therapy, the alternative hypothesis, that the intervention made a difference, is accepted. However, rejecting the null hypothesis does not prove the alternative hypothesis; **rejecting the null only provides a degree of certainty that the null cannot be true given your data**.

Note: Although hypothesis testing provides a reasonable estimate of whether the null hypothesis is true, keep in mind that your calculations will be influenced by the characteristics of the participants in each group, the type of test you use, the number of participants in the study (sample size), and the value you select for representing a statistically significant difference (usually the cut-off value is set at 0.05).

Box 7.1   A Statistician's Perspective: Come Prepared and Meet Early in the Process

You do not need to know a lot about statistics to design a great study. You must, however, **have a clear plan and consult with someone knowledgeable in statistical analyses before you begin a study**. Statisticians are generally happy to offer advice and assist others with data analysis. Statisticians become statisticians because they enjoy analyzing data. It is understandable if you are unsure of which statistical tests to run, which variables to choose, or how to code data in a spreadsheet. These are the types of issues a statistician can advise you about. However, as the investigator, it is your responsibility to develop a good project and you must respect the statistician's time by preparing information and questions before your first meeting.

What to Do:
   Set up a meeting to discuss your project and ask specific questions. A statistician needs to understand your study well enough to offer accurate advice, so come with as much information as you can. At minimum, you need to explain your study question, study groups, primary outcome measure, and all secondary outcome measures. You should provide information on your study sample and how they will be identified. List the information you will record and explain why you are collecting that information.
   Be clear what questions you want to answer with the information you collect. If you are unsure of how best to do something, ask for guidance.
   Meet regularly after the initial consultation to ensure you are collecting and recording information properly.

Early in the process, discuss the statistician's role in the project and agree whether the anticipated work warrants co-authorship on any resulting publications and presentations. If co-authorship is not appropriate, offer to include the statistician in the acknowledgments section of any presentations or publications.

What *Not* to Do:

Do not come with vague ideas about what you want to study and expect the statistician to organize the study for you. Have a plan and ask for guidance, not specific methods.

Do not wait until a study is completed to talk with a statistician. The end of a study is not the time to discover that you should have recorded data as ratio values rather than categorical variables.

Do not expect the statistician to interpret the meaning of your data. Your study question should be well defined before you begin and the interpretation after statistical analysis obvious.

Do not expect the statistician to find something worthwhile in the data set. The statistician cannot go through your data looking for something meaningful. You may have questions about a secondary outcome measure that you would like to analyze further, and it is acceptable to inquire about that. However, searching data to find any result that is statistically significant is never appropriate.

Note: Schedule enough time to discuss the project goals and study design with the statistician.

Tip: If there is no statistician at your institution, contact your former medical school or faculty at a local college or university. Psychology, mathematics, biology, and other science departments often have faculty members who could assist.

Hint: If you are submitting your statistical plans as part of a grant proposal or ethics committee application, do not show up the day before the deadline to ask the statistician what you should include.

CHOOSE ONE-SIDED OR TWO-SIDED HYPOTHESIS TESTS

For most of your studies, you will use **two-sided ("two-tailed") hypothesis tests**. This means you are interested in **results that occur in either direction.** An intervention may increase or decrease the values you measure. For example, an intervention could improve or worsen an outcome. Occupational therapy could decrease the amount of pain medication used, or it could increase the amount used. Two-sided tests are also called **non-directional tests**.

In contrast, **one-sided (one-tailed) hypothesis tests** are called **directional** tests. One-sided tests are used when **measurements only occur in one direction**, or **the investigator is only interested in results in one direction**. For example, in a non-inferiority trial the investigator is only interested in testing if the experimental treatment is no worse than another treatment, not whether it is worse or better.

Note: Investigators should **always use two-sided hypothesis tests unless there is a valid reason to use a one-sided test**. You may suspect that occupational therapy reduces the need for pain medication, but you still must test in both directions.

RECOGNIZE HOW TO REDUCE ERRORS IN STATISTICAL ANALYSIS

Whenever you analyze data, there is a chance you will either find a statistically significant difference among groups when there really is no difference (called a type I error) or, conversely, you will find there is no statistically significant difference among groups when there really is one (type II error). As you plan your project, one of your primary goals is to **design a study that decreases the chance of making either type of error**.

Type I (Alpha) Error

Here, the **null hypothesis is rejected** when it is **true**. With this type of error, the null hypothesis was correct, there is no difference among groups, but your statistical analysis indicated there was a difference. A type I error is also called a **false positive**.

To **reduce the chance of a type I error**, the cut-off level for **significance (alpha)** is set to an acceptable value such as 0.05, meaning there is a 5% chance of committing a type I error for every statistical test you conduct.

There are many factors that influence your chances of getting a type I error, including the significance level (alpha), the number of statistical tests you run, whether any assumptions of statistical tests have been violated, and random chance. The most carefully executed study can still make a type I error simply by collecting data that happen to be extreme.

Note: You should keep the number of statistical tests you run to a minimum, as each test has a chance of making a type I error. When you run several statistical tests on a set of data, you increase your chances of making a type I error in one or more of the tests. Sometimes, statisticians will recommend reducing your significance level below 0.05 (to, for example, 0.01 or even 0.001) to compensate for type I errors compounding over multiple statistical tests.

Type II (Beta) Error

The **null hypothesis is accepted** when it is **false**. This error reflects the failure to reject an untrue null hypothesis, a rather confusing way of stating that your study did not realize the null hypothesis was wrong. With a type II error, there really is a difference among the groups, but no differences were detected. A type II error is also called a **false negative**.

The **power** of the study **reflects the chances of not committing a type II error**. Beta is the chance of making a type II error. Thus, power, defined as 1−beta, estimates the probability a study will be able to detect the true effect of an intervention. Power is often set at 0.80 meaning there is a 20% chance of making a type II error.

The power of a study is influenced by the experimental design, **variance** (variability of each data point from the mean), and sample size. **When sample size** (e.g., the number of participants in the study) **is too small, power decreases and the chances of making a type II error increase**. You are therefore more likely to say there is no difference among groups when there really is one. Thus, underpowered studies *decrease* the likelihood of detecting results that are truly statistically significant.

7.2 DETERMINE AN APPROPRIATE SAMPLE SIZE

To find true differences among groups, the study's sample size must be sufficiently large. Therefore, **investigators must first estimate the number of subjects needed to detect true differences**. The type of data collected influences sample size requirements. For example, measuring dichotomous variables requires more subjects than measuring continuous variables.

Some authors offer **broad guidelines** to use in estimating the sample size. When collecting data from a restricted sample population or completing descriptive studies, such estimates **may provide an indication as to whether you are likely to have enough participants available**. Common advice includes:

- No study with fewer than 30 subjects
- Multiply the number of independent variables by 50, then add 8
- Use 15 subjects per variable
- Use 50 subjects per variable
- Review 10 charts per variable

These guidelines are often helpful to residents trying to decide whether to pursue a project. For example, if a resident is interested in knee surgery outcomes in adolescent athletes aged 13 to 17, she may be able to estimate how many such patients were seen in the past year, based on current patient volumes. If the resident is interested in two variables and estimates there are 45 patients, there may be enough patients for the study. If the resident estimates there are approximately ten patients to evaluate, she might decide to look at additional years, collaborate with another clinic, or revise the study question.

Guidelines provide preliminary information on the likelihood of having a sufficient sample size. However, they are only rough estimates used as a first approximation for the number of subjects needed for a study.

As an investigator, you want to calculate a sample size that is neither too small nor too large (**Box 7.2**). To formally estimate the necessary sample size for

quantitative data, an *a priori* **power analysis** is done. The power analysis estimates the number of subjects needed to achieve statistical significance by assigning values for the **significance level, power,** and **effect size**.

Effect size, as the name suggests, is an index of how large of an "effect" the study finds. Effect size is sometimes confused with significance level (i.e., the p-value) but these are separate things. You can think of **effect size** as the **magnitude of an effect**, whereas the p-**value** reflects the **certainty of the effect**.

Effect sizes are a critical factor in assessing the clinical significance of a study. An intervention may show a statistically significant effect, but this effect, as indicated by the effect size, might be so small that it is clinically insignificant. In clinical research, the **effect size should represent a clinically meaningful difference**. For example, a treatment that reduces the length of hospital stay by 30 minutes is unlikely to be considered clinically meaningful, even if it is statistically significant. However, a treatment that reduces length of hospital stay by 30 hours may be. It is up to the investigators and those to whom the results are communicated to decide whether an effect size is sufficiently large enough to warrant a change in policy or procedure. **Box 7.2** includes some standard guidelines for "small," "medium," and "large" effects.

There are different effect size measures available for different kinds of statistical tests. If you're testing group differences, effect size is generally calculated by dividing the means of each group by the standard deviation of the population from which the groups were taken. To estimate the standard deviation of the population, you can look at data and standard deviations from previous studies on a similar topic or with a similar population. Alternatively, you can do a pilot study to calculate the standard deviation of your population.

In general, a **larger sample size** is better because it has **greater power** and is **more likely to reflect the underlying population.** A larger sample size is also more likely to **detect small differences** among groups. The same study done with a larger sample size might identify differences missed with a smaller sample size. Thus, studies with larger sample sizes are less likely to commit type II errors.

However, there are also concerns if the sample size is too large. **Too large a sample size** may detect small **differences that are not meaningful**. This is because, as the sample size increases, the standard error of the mean decreases, leading small differences to be identified as statistically significant. In addition, an unnecessarily large sample size **uses more resources than needed** and **increases the number of participants** experiencing any **risks** that are associated with the study.

> **Box 7.2   Calculate the Required Sample Size**
>
> 1) Select appropriate statistical tests based on variables and whether one- or two-sided hypothesis testing will be done.
> 2) State the null hypothesis.
> 3) Choose a reasonable, expected effect size for your study based on previous studies.
>   Effect sizes of 0.2 (small), 0.5 (medium) and 0.8 (large) are often used for continuous variables.
> 4) Select alpha and beta levels (by convention alpha 0.05 and beta 0.80, though these should be adjusted as appropriate).
> 5) Use online sample size calculators, such as G*Power, or a published table to determine the desired sample size.
>
> **Note**:   You must estimate some values when calculating sample size. The effect size and variability are usually more difficult to estimate. Consult with an experienced researcher or statistician if you are unsure of how to estimate those.
>
> **Tip**:   Sample size calculators are available (see References and Resources). Note, however, that you must input the correct information, or the recommended sample size will be meaningless.

UNDERSTAND THE DIFFERENT TYPES OF POWER ANALYSES

A power analysis should be done before any study begins. Unfortunately, many new investigators skip this step. Some overlook the importance because they are unfamiliar with how to do the calculation, some believe they will have data to report no matter how many subjects enroll, and others have a limited clinical population to work with and assume power analysis is pointless.

If you know that your subject population is going to be limited, a **compromise power analysis** can be conducted. Instead of using an estimated effect size to determine the number of subjects you will need, a compromise power analysis uses the number of subjects available and estimates what effect size the study will be able to detect. For example, if 45 patient records are available and a compromise power analysis estimates that sample size is enough to detect a medium effect size, and that effect is likely to be clinically meaningful, the study can be justified. Subsequent studies may be necessary, but your project has the potential to provide useful data. However, if you estimate a small effect size that is unlikely to be clinically meaningful, then the study is probably not worth pursuing as designed. **Whenever planning a retrospective chart review, follow best practices (Box 7.3)**.

A **retrospective power analysis** can also be completed on published data to estimate the power of the study or to evaluate the power of an observational study. However, a **retrospective power analysis should not be done after your study is complete to find out if you had enough participants**.

If a power analysis was not done in advance and a study fails to find statistical significance, investigators will not know if there really was no effect of the intervention or whether the study lacked the power to reach statistical significance (i.e., a type II error). Thus, null results are a problem because they are ambiguous and cannot distinguish between these two interpretations. **One way of partially disambiguating a null result is to perform a retrospective power analysis**. A retrospective power analysis will tell you the effect size you could have detected given the number of subjects in your study. If the retrospective power analysis indicates your study was able to detect a large effect size, then you can argue that your findings represent a true negative result, and not a type II error. Of course, doing a power analysis in the beginning is easier and will give others more confidence in your data.

Note: As you increase the number of variables or the number of groups evaluated, you will also need to increase your sample size. Each variable you add to your analysis will decrease your statistical power, making type II errors more likely.

Tip: **The simpler your hypothesis, the easier it will be to interpret your data**. Having one independent and one dependent variable makes data analysis the most straightforward.

Hint: When you know your sample size will be limited, simplify your hypothesis to include only one independent and one dependent variable.

Box 7.3   Retrospective Chart Reviews: Planning Matters (A Lot)

One of the most common study designs in medical research is the retrospective chart review. Investigators answer a question using information already present in patients' medical records (charts). Retrospective chart reviews, although seemingly straightforward, are among the most flawed studies conducted annually and many do not yield useful data. **Unsuccessful studies usually result from a lack of planning, ill-defined study protocols, and a small sample size.**

To succeed, you must **formulate a specific study objective**, determine what information is needed to answer your question, and develop an appropriate protocol that all study team members follow. Like every other study design, you must consider possible obstacles, address weaknesses, define eligibility criteria, and **revise plans until you have a clear and feasible study**.

Stating a vague objective like, "We will review charts for the past 5 years to see how many smokers have heart disease," is not how to begin a chart review. Instead, ask a focused question such as, "Do more smokers have heart disease than non-smokers?"

Then consider what information is necessary to answer that question. First, define what you mean by 'smoker' and 'heart disease'. Are you only interested in those who smoke cigarettes? Do you want to include cigar and pipe smokers too? Are you only studying tobacco smokers, or those who smoke any substance? Are you looking at data from those who currently smoke or anyone who smoked within the past 5 years? Perhaps you define a smoker as anyone who smoked for at least 5 consecutive years within the past 15 years. Will you calculate pack years of smoking history? If so, how?

How will you confirm current or previous smoking status? Is this information consistently listed in the medical record? Is it easy to locate? Will you need to contact patients to get more information? If so, how will that be done and by whom?

What is your definition of heart disease? Are you looking at a history of coronary artery disease, congestive heart failure, valve defects? Will you exclude those with congenital heart disease?

As you consider each element of the study, refine your question, and settle on your **variables**. You may decide, for example, to ask, "Do adults over age 45 who currently smoke at least one pack of cigarettes per week have a higher prevalence of coronary artery disease than those who have not smoked in at least 20 years?"

Next, consider what other information you need from the medical record and why you need it. Will you record gender and age? Age of smoking onset? Patient weight, occupation, family history of heart disease? What diagnoses or medical test results will you record? Why do you need this information and how will it be analyzed? Should you collect information that may be useful for a subsequent study or that could help interpret your primary outcome?

Also think about the logistics of gathering this information, a process called **data abstraction**. Who will pull the information from the records? Who will check eligibility status? Define **data collection** procedures. How will each variable be recorded on the data collection sheet? Who will confirm that data are recorded accurately?

As with any study, you must estimate the sample size needed for statistically meaningful data. Too often, investigators dismiss this step as unnecessary, or reason that they are limited by the number of charts and therefore must settle for what is available. However, you must **always have an estimate of the necessary sample size before you begin**. If you find you need 150 charts but can only access 35 or discover only 56 of the 200 available have all the information you need, the study cannot be completed as planned. **Neglecting sample size calculation is one of the most common reasons chart reviews fail** to produce meaningful data.

Common **best practices** for a successful retrospective chart review include:

1) Define a specific, testable research question.
2) Define the variables to record.
3) Select a sampling method.
4) Define specific inclusion and exclusion criteria.

5) Determine the sample size needed to answer your question.
6) Define how information will be pulled from the records (data abstraction).
7) Define how data will be recorded (data collection).
8) Obtain approval to conduct the study from Institutional Review Board or ethics committee.

Note: To limit the sample size needed, develop a focused question with few variables.

Tip: Complete a pilot study to confirm that the charts contain the information you seek, and that your data collection methods are appropriate. Get IRB approval before you begin any pilot study.

Hint: Review pilot data for inter- and intra-rater variability and revise protocols and training as necessary.

Remember: Before you embark on a retrospective chart review, frame a testable question that can be answered with information *consistently* listed in the medical record.

7.3 AVOID "FISHING" FOR STATISTICAL SIGNIFICANCE
The practice of analyzing every possible variable in the data set, with the goal of finding something that will come out as statistically significant, is commonly referred to as a "statistical fishing expedition." This usually occurs when the primary outcome fails to produce the expected, or "desired," result anticipated by the investigator. Such investigators are hoping that with enough effort, statistically significant results will show up somewhere. This is, of course, a terrible idea, as any statistician will tell you.

Every additional variable an investigator analyzes with inferential statistics increases the chance of a type I error (false positive). Thus, if you run enough statistical tests, eventually something is likely to turn up as statistically significant simply because some of the data happen to be a little extreme. When "fishing" for statistical significance, the probability of a type I error becomes so high it is virtually inevitable. It is much better to limit the analysis to a few pre-determined tests of the key hypothesis and report a lack of statistical significance when that is what the results indicate.

Of course, there are situations in which multiple statistical tests are required to fully examine the hypothesis in question. Fortunately, there are several ways to reduce the type I error rate in these circumstances, such as making the significance level much more conservative (rejecting the null hypothesis at 0.01 instead of 0.05, for example). The statistician on the project can assist in determining the best course of action in such cases.

Hint: Investigators should avoid the mindset of "hoping" for certain results. Research seeks to identify truths, not outcomes that appeal to the investigators.

Remember: Your hypothesis must be stated in advance, not created during or after data are collected.

7.4 CHOOSE STATISTICAL APPROACHES THAT FIT YOUR STUDY DESIGN

The following summaries provide a starting point for choosing the appropriate statistical tests for your data. Several books and online resources illustrate decision trees that are helpful in determining which tests are suitable for your study design and variables (see also Resources and References).

STATISTICAL APPROACHES BASED ON STUDY TYPE

Descriptive Observational Studies (*Case Report, Case Series, Descriptive Cross-Sectional Study*):
  Use: *Descriptive statistics* (e.g., mean, median, range, variance, frequency distribution); *prevalence* (cross-sectional study).

Analytical Observational Studies (*Analytical Cross-Sectional, Case-Control, Cohort Studies*):
  Use: *Inferential Statistics, risk ratio, odds ratio, relative risk, absolute risk, prevalence, incidence,* and *descriptive statistics,* as appropriate.
  Analytical Cross-Sectional Studies: *Inferential statistics, odds ratio*
  Case-Control Studies: *Inferential statistics, odds ratio, relative risk, prevalence* (retrospective studies), *incidence* (concurrent studies).
  Cohort Studies: *Inferential statistics, relative risk, absolute risk, incidence* (prospective studies).

Experimental studies (*Controlled Trials, Randomized Controlled Trials*):
  Use: *Inferential statistics, risk ratio, odds ratio, relative risk, absolute risk, prevalence, incidence,* and *descriptive statistics,* as appropriate.

STATISTICAL TESTS BASED ON TYPE AND DISTRIBUTION OF VARIABLES

Categorical Variables

Larger sample size	Chi-squared test
Smaller sample size	Fisher exact test

Tip: If any of the responses are fewer than five or the sum of all cells in your contingency table are less than 50, consider the sample size is small.

Continuous Variables

  Parametric Tests: Use for continuous variables that are **normally distributed**.
  Non-Parametric Tests: Use for continuous variables that are **not normally distributed** (skewed) or **smaller sample sizes** (e.g., less than 30).

Frequently Used Methods

Type of Analysis	Parametric Tests Used	Non-parametric Tests Used
Compare two groups		
Unpaired	Unpaired *t*-test	Mann–Whitney *U* test
Paired	Paired *t*-test	Wilcoxon signed rank test
Compare three or more groups		
One outcome	Analysis of variance (ANOVA)	Kruskal–Wallis test
Establish associations	Pearson's correlation coefficient	Spearman's rho correlation coefficient

Other Common Methods

Type of Analysis	Parametric Tests Used	Non-Parametric Tests Used
Compare three or more groups		
Repeated observations/participant	Repeated measures ANOVA	Friedman's test
Multiple dependent variables	Multivariate analysis of variance (MANOVA)	
Covariate analysis	Analysis of covariance (ANCOVA)	
Make predictions		
One predictor variable	Simple regression	Kendall–Theil regression
Two or more predictor variables	Multiple/logistic regression	

7.5 CONCLUSIONS

During the study design phase, you determine which statistical tests are appropriate for the variables you are evaluating. You also estimate the sample size needed to produce meaningful results. Consultation with a statistician should occur prior to beginning the study to ensure all necessary data are collected and recorded in a manner appropriate for answering the research question.

APPENDIX A: TERMS AND CONCEPTS ASSOCIATED WITH STATISTICAL TESTS

VARIABLES

Independent variables (predictor variables) are those properties thought to cause a change in other variables. In clinical research, these are often called **exposures**, **interventions**, or **risk factors**.

Dependent variables occur due to changes to an independent variable. These are the variables that are **observed** or **measured** in a study. Dependent variables are the **outcomes** or **diseases** identified in clinical research.

Categorical variables have **no numerical value**. They are assigned to a finite number of groups or categories and can be either **qualitative** or **quantitative**. Categorical variables may be dichotomous, nominal, or ordinal.

> **Dichotomous** (or binary) variables are placed into **two groups** without any intrinsic order or ranking
> *Examples: male/female; yes/no; right/left*

> **Nominal** variables are assigned to more than two groups
> *Examples: ethnicity; occupation*
> **Ordinal** variables are ordered or ranked within two or more groups.
> *Examples: rank pain scores 0–10; satisfaction score 1–5*

Continuous variables are associated with a numerical value. Continuous variables may be intervals or ratios.

> **Interval** variables are measured along a continuum, have **constant equal difference** between two values, but **do not** have a **true 0 measurement**.
> *Examples: IQ scores, pH value*

> **Ratio** variables have a **true 0 value**. The 0 value represents an absence of the variable.
> *Example: on the Kelvin scale, 0 represents a complete absence of heat.*

MEASURES

P-values are calculated to determine the probability of finding a difference as large, or larger, by chance. Often set at 0.05 meaning there is a 5% chance that the finding was random.

Confidence levels are used to determine the probability that a population parameter, such as the mean, will fall between two values. Confidence intervals are often set at 95% indicating there is a 95% chance the true value falls within the range identified.

Odds ratio: The relative chance an outcome will occur from a given exposure.

Relative risk: The ratio of the probability of an outcome occurring in an exposed group to the probability of an outcome occurring in an unexposed group.

Absolute risk: The odds of an outcome occurring during a defined period.

Prevalence: An indication of how frequent an outcome is in a population; the *total* number of cases of a disease at any time.

Incidence: The number of *new* cases in a specified period.

REFERENCES AND RESOURCES

BOOKS

Elmore JG, Wild D, Nelson HD, Katz DL. *Jekel's Epidemiology, Biostatistics, Preventive Medicine, and Public Health.* 5th ed. St. Louis: Elsevier; 2020.

Ferguson, CJ. An effect size primer: A guide for clinicians and researchers. In: AE Kazdin eds. *Methodological Issues and Strategies in Clinical Research.* 4th ed. Washington, DC: American Psychological Association; 2016.

Herzog MH, Francis G, Clarke A. *Understanding Statistics and Experimental Design. How to Not Lie with Statistics.* Cham: Springer; 2019.

Kapur K. Principles of biostatistics. In: Robertson D and Williams GH eds. *Clinical and Translational Science.* 2nd ed. London: Elsevier; 2017.

ARTICLES

Andrade C. Understanding relative risk, odds ratio, and related terms: As simple as it can get. *J Clin Psychiatry.* 2015;76(7):e857–e861.

Button KS. Statistical rigor and the perils of chance. *eNeuro.* 2016;3(4):0030–16.2016.

Charan J, Biswas T. How to calculate sample size for different study designs in medical research. *Indian J Psychol Med.* 2013;35(2):121–126.

Faul, F, Erdfelder, E, Lang, A-G, Buchner, A. G*Power 3: A flexible statistical power analysis for the social, behavioral, and biomedical sciences. *Behav Res Methods.* 2007;39:175–191.

Neideen T, Brasel K. Understanding statistical tests. *J Surg Educ.* 2007;64(2):93–96.

Vetter TR, Mascha EJ. Defining the primary outcomes and justifying secondary outcomes of a study: Usually, the fewer, the better. *Anesth Analg.* 2017;125(2):678–681.

Vetter TR, Mascha EJ. Bias, confounding, and interaction: Lions and Tigers, and Bears, Oh My! *Anesth Analg.* 2017;125(3):1042–1048.

Wang X, Ji X. Sample size estimation in clinical research: From randomized controlled trials to observational studies. *Chest.* 2020;158(1S):S12–S20.

RESOURCES

POWER ANALYSIS
G*Power calculator

G*Power is a free, open-source tool for power analysis.

- https: www.psychologie.hhu.de/arbeitsgruppen/allgemeine-psychologie
  -und-arbeitspsychologie/gpower

STATISTICAL SOFTWARE
JASP is a free, open-source statistical package from the University of Amsterdam.

- https://jasp-stats.org/

STATISTICAL DECISION TREE EXAMPLES

- https://www.slideserve.com/zitomira-pascha/statistical-decision-tree
- https://cursa.ihmc.us/rid=1282073589603_785092654_146/Data%20Analysis%20Tree.cmap

Research with Human Subjects: Preparing an Application for the Institutional Review Board

Lynne M. Bianchi, Ph.D., Joyce Babyak, Ph.D., and Robert Maholic, D.O.

Tips for Success:

> Write your Institutional Review Board (IRB) application for a diverse audience whose focus is protecting the rights and safety of participants.
> Include all necessary information in sufficient detail so IRB members understand exactly what the study involves.

Warnings:

> A poorly prepared application lacking necessary information will be sent back with questions you must address before the IRB considers whether to approve your application.
> Having to address questions delays your study start date.

Key Concept: The materials you prepare for your IRB application can be used in other documents.

Any research involving human subjects requires oversight from an ethics committee, such as the **Institutional Review Board** (IRB) found at most universities and hospitals in the United States (U.S.). Ethics committees are charged with protecting human subjects from any harm, including loss of confidentiality, undue coercion, and physical or mental suffering. Every research study with human subjects must be submitted to the IRB for review and **written approval must be obtained prior to initiating a study**. Even if a project is deemed minimal risk, failure to contact the IRB is a serious matter.

Because most physicians are ethical individuals who truly care about their patients and work tirelessly to prevent any harm, they could never imagine treating a patient in a manner that could damage health or violate confidentiality. To these physicians, it may seem unnecessary, a bit insulting, and rather frustrating to have to fill out, in great detail, forms that explain precisely what one will and will not do with subjects during a research study.

DOI: 10.1201/9781003126478-8

Such frustrations are particularly common for investigators conducting low-risk observational studies or chart reviews. However, **even the most ethical individuals have biases, make mistakes, and overlook ways they put participants at risk**. For example, an investigator may unintentionally include or exclude some patients from a study, use a research assistant who does not have proper training, or fail to secure a data sheet with patient demographics.

For studies that involve more than minimal risk, the IRB weighs the potential risks and potential benefits, evaluates the investigator's plans to minimize the risks, and assesses the procedures to address any adverse events. Any concerns are addressed prior to approving and implementing the study. Thus, an ethics committee **ensures subjects are properly protected** and **limits the likelihood that investigators will make unintentional errors**.

This chapter describes the elements of the IRB review process, levels of participant risk, and the information commonly included in an IRB application. Although the focus is on IRB policies, the basic elements will be the same for all ethics committees that review research involving human subjects.

Preparing materials to submit to the IRB, while perhaps frustrating at the time, it actually very useful. As discussed later in this chapter, **most of the text you prepare for the IRB is used in other documents**, such as grant applications and manuscripts. Recognizing the benefits of well-prepared documents will alleviate the sense that you are "wasting time" preparing an application for the IRB.

8.1 COMPLETE REQUIRED TRAINING

Before engaging in any research project involving human subjects, all investigators must receive appropriate training regarding the rules and regulations governing research with human subjects and understand why they are so important. Box 8.1 reviews the origins and bases of human subjects' protections that form the foundation of current IRB regulations.

In the U.S., investigators, co-investigators, and research assistants often obtain training online *via* the **Collaborative Institutional Training Initiative** (CITI). The CITI program offers several online courses to teach investigators essential principles of working with human subjects, including topics related to investigator responsibilities and participant rights and protections. In addition to the core training modules, there are specific modules for principal investigators, co-investigators, IRB members, and those using clinical devices and investigational drugs. CITI also offers courses in animal care and use for investigators who work with animal models. CITI training certification is valid for three or four years, depending on the module, after which refresher courses are required. Institutions often purchase an annual subscription for these courses. Courses can also be purchased by individuals.

The U.S. Office for Human Research Protections (OHRP) offers a **Human Protections Training course**, consisting of four lessons. These are free online training modules that may be used at some institutions.

If your institution requires CITI or OHRP training modules, your IRB administrator will tell you how to access the system, which modules to complete, and how to document successful completion.

Training is also important for you to recognize and appreciate the differences between experimental practice and experimental research. Experimental medical research involves *groups* of patients receiving defined interventions. However, trying different interventions during *routine care of a single* patient is not considered research. Be sure you know the differences between practice, experimentation, and research (**Box 8.2**).

Note: Complete all required training *before* you assist in any way with any project, including helping a colleague with chart reviews or data analysis.

Tip: For those interested in research using animal models, see **Box 8.4**.

**Box 8.1   Foundations of Current Ethical Guidelines
for Human Subjects Research**

Current guidelines and regulations for research involving human subjects have evolved over time largely in response to unethical practices. Some of the studies leading to the need for Institutional Review Board (IRB) oversight were intended to advance medical knowledge, highlighting how easily practices become harmful to participants and society when not guided by established principles. The practices that led to the need for IRBs are rightly seen as shocking. However, those unethical practices were conducted within the past 100 years by educated physicians and health care professionals, a sober reminder that unethical practices can develop at any time in any setting.

The **Nuremberg Code** established the first guidelines for conducting medical research. The Nuremberg Code stemmed from Nazi experimentation on prisoners held in concentration camps during World War II. Prior to the Nuremberg Code, there were no established regulations for medical experimentation on human subjects and therefore the need for clear international guidelines was recognized. In 1948, the World Medical Association's **Declaration of Geneva** incorporated the ten principles of the Nuremberg Code and further emphasized the ethical responsibilities of physicians in protecting patients' safety and rights. The **Declaration of Helsinki** expanded on the principles of the Nuremberg Code and together these became the foundation of the international guidelines used today.

The **Nuremberg Code** (1947) specified ten basic principles to guide all research with humans. Key elements include:

- Voluntary consent must be obtained from all participants.
- Participants can withdraw from a study at any time.
- Studies must avoid unnecessary physical or mental injury or suffering to participants.
- A study must be based on previous knowledge that justifies its need.
- An experiment must have benefits for society.
- Any risk to participants must be justified.
- No study should be conducted if death or disabling injury is likely to occur.
- Procedures to limit risks need to be in place.
- Investigators must be qualified personnel.
- Investigators must be willing to stop a study if continuation is likely to result in harm.

The **Declaration of Helsinki** (1964) provided further guidelines for properly documenting research data, protecting participant privacy, and obtaining consent from participants or a legally authorized representative. The Declaration has been modified several times to include clarifications and additional protections. In addition to the core principles first outlined in the Nuremberg Code, the Declaration of Helsinki notes:

- Physicians have a duty to safeguard patients and to protect the health, privacy, and dignity of research subjects.
- Informed consent must include information on the study aims, methods, benefits, potential risks, or discomforts.
- Research methods must be designed to ensure adherence to proper research ethics, an acceptable risk-to-benefit ratio must exist, and investigators must stop a study if the risks are found to outweigh the benefits.
- Extreme care should be taken regarding the use of placebo; placebo treatments are to be used only in the absence of an existing proven therapy.

The need for additional safeguards became apparent when the practices surrounding the **United States Tuskegee Study of Untreated Syphilis in the Negro Male** (1930s–1970s) were revealed. The study was initiated to observe the natural course of syphilis. However, the men were not told the purpose of the study, or informed if they tested positive for syphilis. Further, when penicillin was found to be an effective treatment in the 1940s, the medication was never offered to the men in the study. The study continued for 40 years until someone finally brought the unethical practices to public attention. The practices surrounding this study led to the **Belmont Report** (1978) and federal **laws requiring Institutional Review Boards** (IRBs) to oversee human subjects' research.

The Belmont Report highlights the importance of respect for persons, beneficence, and justice in research studies and expands requirements regarding acceptable practices for obtaining informed consent.

Respect for Persons centers on the capacity for human beings to make autonomous decisions. For example, informed consent is a practice designed to show respect for an individual's right to make decisions about his body and health care. When individuals are not capable of making these decisions, respect is honored by provisions to ensure that they are protected and, in some cases, have a proxy make decisions for them.

In clinical research, **respect for persons** is demonstrated by ensuring the following for each person being asked to participate in a study:

- Consent to participate is voluntary and informed.
- Subject has the right to withdraw from participation without penalty.
- Subject's privacy and confidentiality are protected.

Further, the Belmont Report provides special protections for those with diminished autonomy, such as children, prisoners, and those who are cognitively impaired.

Beneficence maximizes benefits, minimizes harms, and asks investigators to consider whether participants are treated in a way they would wish to be treated. Beneficence requires:

- A study to be designed to minimize risks and maximize potential benefits.
- Any risks to be justified by the potential benefits to the individual and/ or society.
- Conflicts of interest to be minimized and documented to limit bias in judgments related to research conduct.

Justice requires the fair selection of subjects, so the risks and benefits of the research burden are evenly distributed among eligible participants across society. This is achieved by ensuring:

- Participants are selected for reasons directly related to the problem studied.
- A research study does not systematically select any group of individuals simply due to ease of availability or compromised position.
- A research study does not systematically exclude a group of individuals for whom the results are likely to be applied.

Informed consent, which is directly related to respect for persons, as noted above, must include descriptions of the procedures, purposes, risks, and benefits associated with participation in the study and any alternative procedures available.

- The language in the consent document must be written to be understandable by the participant.
- Consent must be voluntary and requested without coercion or undue influence.
- If participants, such as children, are not capable of giving fully informed consent for themselves, informed consent on their behalf must be received from an appropriate proxy, often termed a legally authorized representative, such as a parent or legal guardian.

Note: Chapter 9 reviews elements required for informed consent.

8.2 UNDERSTAND THE SERIOUSNESS OF VIOLATING ANY REGULATION

Many of the studies conducted during residency will be minimal or low risk, yet the IRB still needs to review your plans and ensure that your procedures meet all requirements. Each IRB is governed by the rules of the OHRP, a division of the U.S. Department of Health and Human Services. **Failure to follow IRB regulations can lead to serious consequences for the investigators and their institution**, such as citations and other consequences, based on the nature of the violation.

All citations are **posted on the public OHRP website**, including non-compliance violations for an IRB that fails to properly review projects or maintain adequate records. No investigator, IRB, or institution wants to be listed on that website.

While you may feel confident you would never endanger participants in any of your studies, you might overlook other regulations that lead to citations. For example, failure to contact the IRB and receive approval prior to implementing an anonymous, minimal-risk survey to fellow residents is reason for a citation.

Note: Any citation can prevent future research and funding opportunities for you, your co-investigators, or your institution.

Remember: All investigators, including **resident research assistants**, are **responsible for notifying the IRB regarding any concerns about patient rights or safety,** including knowledge of a study being conducted without IRB approval.

Box 8.2   When Experimentation Does Not Meet the Definition of Research

Research may use experimental approaches, but experimentation that occurs during routine medical practice is usually not a form of research.

When patients choose to join a research study, they participate to help investigators evaluate a treatment or approach. In some cases, participation in a research study benefits individual patients, but the purpose of the study is to produce generalizable knowledge, not to offer treatment to individuals. Participation in a research study therefore differs from what occurs during medical practice.

Practice: Unlike research, practice "refers to a class of activities designed solely to enhance the well-being of an individual patient or client. The purpose of medical or behavioral practice is to provide diagnosis, preventative treatment or therapy … with a reasonable chance of success" (Levine 1981, 2). Activities that constitute medical practice are not under the purview of the IRB.

Experimentation: Medical practice often involves some forms of experimentation with patients, whether to determine a diagnosis or identify an intervention that will successfully treat a specific patient. Because the purpose in each case is to benefit a particular patient, this activity, even when it involves experimentation of some kind, is not considered research.

Thus, when specific interventions are forms of practice, even if they involve some degree of individualized experimentation, they do not fall under the IRB. However, it is possible for research and practice to be conducted together. For example, a research study may evaluate the safety of a particular practice. As the Belmont Report notes, "the general rule is that if there is any element of research in an activity, that activity should undergo review for the protection of human subjects" (1979, Part A).

It may seem unnecessary to explain the differences between medical practice experimentation and research experimentation, but it is essential for you as a physician to understand these differences to avoid inadvertently crossing the boundary of acceptable practice.

Hint: Whenever you are unsure if treatment or diagnostic procedures include a research component, consult the IRB.

8.3 FOLLOW BEST PRACTICES FOR RESEARCH AND QUALITY IMPROVEMENT PROJECTS

Two types of investigations are common in clinical practice: research studies and quality improvement projects. Although both involve gathering and analyzing data, they serve different purposes and are reviewed by different committees. The IRB is charged with protecting human subjects involved in research studies.

NOTE THE PURPOSE AND PROCEDURES ASSOCIATED WITH RESEARCH STUDIES AND QUALITY IMPROVEMENT PROJECTS

Research studies involve **systematic evaluation** and are intended to develop or contribute to **generalizable knowledge**. Data are collected with the intention of disseminating the findings beyond the department or division of an institution. Most are developed with the intention of publishing or presenting the data to an audience outside of the institution. Systematic evaluations completed as part of educational training, regardless of whether they are disseminated outside the institution, are also classified as research studies.

In contrast, **quality improvement (QI)** or **quality assurance (QA)** projects are designed to **evaluate an internal process**. These studies assess existing processes, without manipulating any variables. There is **no risk to participants** as standard of care is provided. In addition, investigators have access to all data as part of their professional responsibilities. To be considered QI/QA projects, the study must not infringe on patient privacy, breach patient confidentiality, nor pose any risk to patients or staff. The intent of these projects is to share the information with the institution to improve processes or procedures. Although some studies are ultimately presented or published for audiences interested in QI/QA issues, the primary purpose is not to disseminate the findings widely.

Most institutions have separate committees that review research and QI/QA projects. When necessary, consult with the appropriate committee(s) at your institution to determine the type of review required for a proposed project.

Note: IRB oversight is usually not required for oral history projects nor for some types of observational field work that do not meet the definition of research. Though less common in medical research, if your project appears to meet such criteria, consult with your IRB administrator to determine if IRB oversight is required.

8.4 UNDERSTAND IRB REVIEW PROCESSES

As an investigator, you should know how your IRB or ethics committee functions and be familiar with the regulations developed to protect those who participate in your research studies. You will learn much of this material through CITI training.

IRBs in the U.S. follow the rules and regulations of the Department of Health and Human Services (HHS) available through the Office for Human Research Protections (OHRP; https://www.hhs.gov/ohrp).

Human subject protections are part of the **Code of Federal Regulations (CFR)** 45, part 46 (45 CFR 46). These regulations are divided into four subparts to address different areas of human subjects' protections. **Subpart A**, referred to as the "**Common Rule**," details requirements for IRB membership and deliberations, informed consent, and the Assurances of Compliance for institutions with IRBs. **Subpart B** addresses additional protections for pregnant women, human fetuses, and neonates; **subpart C** explains additional protections for prisoners, while **subpart D** details additional protections for children.

The IRB evaluates all studies following OHRP policies. Necessary **materials submitted to the IRB** typically include an **application form**, a narrative description of the research procedures (**protocol**), the **data collection tool**, and, where applicable, the **consent form** and **recruitment document**.

Note: Consent is generally required unless study design and specific criteria indicate that a waiver to informed consent is appropriate. Consent may be waived, for example, for some retrospective chart reviews or studies analyzing existing biospecimens (see Appendix B). Only your IRB can determine if a waiver of consent is acceptable for your study.

NOTE HOW LEVEL OF RISK INFLUENCES *IRB* REVIEW
The IRB reviews studies using one of three mechanisms: **full committee** (quorum), **expedited**, or **exempt**. The type of review depends on several criteria including the **study design** (observational or experimental), the **information collected** (e.g., standard educational tests, sensitive questions, medical history), the population studied (e.g., children, adults, prisoners, pregnant women), and the **level of risk to participants** (no more than minimal risk, minimal risk, or greater than minimal risk). In all cases, the IRB must make determinations about review category and application requirements consistent with OHRP regulations.

One key criterion for determining the level of review is whether the study puts participants at greater than minimal risk. **Minimal risk is defined as "the probability and magnitude of harm or discomfort anticipated in the research are not greater in and of themselves than those ordinarily encountered in daily life or during the performance of routine physical or psychological examinations or tests."** Note, however, that even though some risks may not be severe in nature, if they are outside those encountered in routine examinations or everyday life, those risks are categorized as more than minimal risk.

Full Committee (Quorum) Review

Full committee (quorum) review is required for studies that are **more than minimal risk**; studies that involve **physical or psychological harm greater than occurs in everyday life or during routine examinations or tests**. Randomized control trials or other experimental studies often fall under this category. In addition, common procedures that would not be included as part of standard care, such as a study that requires a blood sample that would not otherwise be drawn, may fall under full committee review. Many projects involving children, prisoners, or other vulnerable populations require full committee review unless they meet the established criteria for another category of review.

For the full committee review process, members of the IRB discuss your application at a **convened meeting**. These meetings are held at regularly scheduled times, often on a monthly or bi-monthly basis, depending on the size of the institution and the number of applications received. Committee members receive your application in advance, allowing them time to evaluate your project and note any areas of concern to discuss at the meeting. At the convened meeting, committee members discuss any issues or questions they have about the application. Many institutions require the principal investigator (PI) to present a brief overview of the study and answer questions from panel members. After the presentation, the PI leaves and the IRB discusses the application.

Decisions: The committee may approve the application as submitted, require modifications, request additional information, or disapprove the project. Many times, the committee will request clarifications before making a final decision. The IRB chairperson or administrator compiles the agreed upon recommendations to share with the PI. Any required changes are submitted back to the IRB for further consideration. A project cannot begin until the revised application receives written approval.

Note: Although a single activity may not be associated with significant risk, if it is outside the standard of care, the IRB must evaluate if those risks, especially in combination with any other study procedures, are acceptable.

Expedited Review

Expedited review is used when studies involve **minimal risk** and **meet specific federal criteria** (see Appendix A). The IRB chairperson or administrator determines whether a project is eligible for expedited review. With an expedited review process, a **subset of IRB members reviews** your project, **without a convened meeting**. Because projects in this category do not require the full committee to discuss your application, the review process may take less time.

Examples of projects that may fall under the expedited review category are those that collect voice recordings for research purposes, non-invasive collection of biological specimens for research purposes (e.g., nail clippings, mucosal cells *via* buccal swab), or use of approved medical devices as intended.

Materials submitted for an expedited review are the same as for full committee review and generally include the application form, protocol, data collection tool, and applicable consent and recruitment forms.

The expedited review process may also be used to **approve minor changes to a previously approved project**, such as addition of another qualified investigator or extending the duration of an approved project.

Decisions: IRB members evaluating an application *via* expedited review may approve a project as submitted, request additional information, require modifications, or request full committee review if they feel additional discussion or perspectives are warranted. Applications under expedited review cannot be disapproved. Any applications that are not approved through the expedited review process go to the full committee.

Note: Should you think the IRB is picky (and you will think this at times), remember that committee members must pay attention to the "specific federal criteria." As an example of what is listed under criteria qualifying for expedited review:

> Collection of blood samples by finger stick, heel stick, ear stick, or venipuncture as follows:
>
> a) from healthy non-pregnant adults who weigh at least 110 pounds. For these subjects, the amounts drawn may not exceed 550 ml in an 8-week period and collection may not occur more frequently than 2 times per week; or
>
> b) from other adults and children, considering the age, weight, and health of the subjects, the collection procedure, the amount of blood to be collected, and the frequency with which it will be collected. For these subjects the amount drawn may not exceed the lesser of 50 ml or 3 ml per kg [kilogram] in an 8-week period and collection may not occur more frequently than 2 times per week.

Before submitting your application, check the criteria for expedited review and explain all relevant information clearly so it is apparent that your study fits in this category. You can consult the OHRP.gov website or contact your IRB for current expedited review criteria (see also Appendix A). As with every IRB application, the IRB ultimately determines the appropriate category of review.

Exempt from IRB Review and Oversight

Exempt from IRB committee review and oversight applies to projects with **no more than minimal risk** that **meet specific criteria**. The IRB chairperson or administrator determines whether a project is eligible for exemption from review and oversight. Examples of studies that may qualify for exemption include research evaluating normal educational practices and surveys of non-sensitive topics administered to adult subjects.

The primary differences in review procedures for the exempt category and the other categories are (1) the IRB administrator or committee chairperson can review the application to determine exemption status, and (2) exempt studies are not subject to continuing (annual) review.

An application requesting exemption is often shorter and the review process is streamlined compared with the other types of review; however, because these studies involve human subjects, **investigators must maintain the same ethical standards and complete the same training** as for other categories of IRB review.

Decisions: If the application is complete and the study procedures meet the standards for exemption from committee review, the investigator will receive written notification that the project is exempt from IRB review and the project may begin. Just as with a full committee or expedited review process, **a study cannot begin until written notification is received from the IRB**.

If the study does not meet the criteria for exemption, the IRB will inform the investigators which review mechanism to use.

Important Note: **An investigator *cannot* determine that a study is exempt.** Only the IRB can determine if a study is exempt from committee review and IRB oversight.

Tip: In most cases, you will **submit two documents to the IRB**: an **application form** and the **protocol**, the narrative description of your project. **Readers should be able to follow each separately**; do not expect IRB members to flip between the two to identify the relevant information needed to understand your study procedures. Before submission, confirm that **all information is consistent in application and protocol**.

Hint: Some institutions will not require a separate protocol for an exemption request, but investigators should create a written protocol for team members to follow.

Recognize Why IRB Membership Is Diverse

Diversity is needed in IRB committee membership to represent various perspectives and areas of expertise. This diversity helps ensure all aspects of the project are thoughtfully considered and properly evaluated. IRBs are comprised of at least five members including at least one scientist, one non-scientist, and one member not affiliated with the institution, often a member of the community. Committee members consider the perspective of participants, participant safety, and the scientific integrity of the study. Most committees will have more than the minimal number of required members to ensure broad expertise and multiple viewpoints.

Scientists include trained physicians, nurses, other health care providers, and lab researchers. These panel members have the appropriate training and expertise to understand the scientific background of the study, proposed procedures, and potential risks to participants. Larger institutions often include several scientists to cover a range of specializations. These members evaluate the scientific procedures as well as the ethical treatment of participants.

Non-scientists often include members of the community in which the study takes place and ethicists. These IRB members contribute important perspectives from outside the field of scientific research and improve the review process in several ways. For example, the presence of at least one non-scientist requires the materials be free of overly technical language and medical jargon. This sometimes brings to light concerns that might otherwise go unnoticed. Community members bring a perspective shaped by their community. While no individual can truly represent the entire community, these members are often attuned to risks and benefits associated with a study in ways other panel members are not.

The training of ethicists gives them a deep understanding of the three key principles: respect for persons, beneficence, and justice, and related concepts and practices, as well as the way these principles may be honored or challenged by the totality of the proposed study. To appreciate the significance of non-scientists on the IRB, imagine if community members and ethicists were invited to review the Tuskegee Study.

Because of the diverse membership of an IRB, you must prepare your application so that it can be understood by every member of the committee. **Do not write your applications as if all reviewers are experienced physicians in your specialty area**. Assume those reading your application and protocol are unfamiliar with the topic and methods you are describing. Write so your study can be understood by a non-scientist community member, a scientist outside the medical field, an ethicist, and your department chair. This is true whether your application is reviewed by full committee, expedited, or exempt procedures.

All IRB members will find your documents are easier to comprehend and evaluate when you write for a non-expert. Experts in your field will not be offended if you define a term or explain a procedure they know. However, non-experts will become confused and frustrated if they cannot follow what you are describing. Ultimately, any **lack of clarity will lead to questions from the committee and delays in IRB approval**.

Tip: Try to read your application from a reviewer's perspective. Double check that all information is provided in a clear and concise manner and that the information is placed in the appropriate sections.

Remember: The easier your documents are to follow, the sooner your IRB application will be approved.

Include All Necessary Information in the IRB Application
Each institution has its own IRB application forms and submission procedures. The information you submit will depend in part on the type of study, the subject population, and whether consent is required. You will need to contact your

IRB administrator or your institution's IRB website for current forms and submission requirements.

Your institution's application form will likely include these common elements:

Study Title, Personnel, and Contact Information

The title should reflect the purpose of the study. This title will also be included on the consent forms and should be comprehensible to those outside the medical field. Personnel include the principal investigator (PI) and any co-investigators, research assistants, study coordinators, or data analysts. The PI will need to confirm that all study personnel have completed the training required by your institution (e.g., CITI modules). Contact information listed should be work addresses, phone numbers, and emails.

Study Purpose

This section gives a brief overview of why your study is being conducted and lists the specific aims of the proposed study. The study objectives or hypotheses are clearly stated so reviewers know what information you seek.

Background Literature and Preliminary Data

This section explains why your study is needed and how it will address unanswered questions that are important and relevant to your field of study. You will describe current knowledge based on existing literature and any preliminary data you have collected.

Note: You must have IRB approval to collect preliminary data from human subjects. Thus, even pilot studies must be reviewed and approved before you can begin data collection.

Study Design and Study Population

You will describe the study design you will use, indicate primary and secondary outcomes measured, the total number of subjects needed for the study, the results of your power analysis or other appropriate means for determining adequate sample size, and the statistical analyses you plan to use at the completion of the study. You will also list and justify participant inclusion and exclusion criteria.

Research Activities

This section explains everything that occurs from the initial screening of potential subjects to final follow-up assessments. The duration of subject participation and the estimated time for participants to complete each aspect of the study are indicated. Descriptions of any tasks, surveys, questionnaires, or evaluations the participants will complete are included. You will attach copies of these materials with your application.

Hint: Make sure your descriptions are detailed and clear so reviewers can assess participant risk for *each* activity.

Risks and Benefits

The IRB completes a risk/benefit assessment for every study to decide whether potential risks are outweighed by potential benefits. The issues to consider vary with each study. For example, the considerations in a risk/benefit assessment evaluating potential side effects of a new medication that may treat an otherwise incurable disease are quite different from those involving a prospective study comparing two established physical therapy interventions.

Risks range from the loss of confidentiality to severe adverse events related to an experimental procedure. You will **include all the potential risks, discomforts, or inconveniences a participant may experience**. You will indicate the **steps taken to minimize** those risks, discomforts, or inconveniences, as well as how you will protect participant privacy. You will also **address risks that may occur should a participant withdraw from the study** and what steps will be taken to limit those risks. You will include descriptions of financial risks, such as any research-related costs to individuals, and how you would address any clinically significant adverse event that might occur.

A **benefit** refers to something that occurs as part of the study intervention that directly impacts a single participant in a positive way. In many studies, there will be no direct benefits to participants, or it will be unclear if there is a benefit. For example, when testing a new medication that may improve a medical condition, it is not yet known if the medication provides a benefit over standard care.

Do not try to make a benefit where one does not exist. If there are no benefits, state there are no known direct benefits to participants. Indicating that a participant may feel good about participating in a study, even if true, is not a direct benefit. Sometimes, participants receive additional medical care or services as part of a study, which are usually considered to be indirect benefits and may be included in the study description but are not a direct benefit resulting from the study intervention. There is generally no need to include a statement that the study may benefit future patients or society as those benefits are not known and do not directly impact those who participate.

If you are unclear on how to describe potential benefits or risks for your study, contact your IRB administrator or chairperson for further instruction.

Compensation and Incentives

Your study may reimburse participants for gas mileage, parking fees, or provide a small stipend or gift card for participating. Your study may pay for additional medical tests related to the study. You will describe any compensation or incentives and indicate when they will be given to participants.

It is usually acceptable to offer some compensation or small incentive for participating, but the value cannot be so large as to induce someone to participate in a study they would otherwise decline. Furthermore, because participants have a right to withdraw from a study at any time, it must be clear that the incentive does not coerce someone to remain in the study.

When deciding what incentive to offer, consider the perspective of potential participants. For example, your opinion of the influence of a $50 gift card may be different from that of another person.

Consent Process and Consent Forms

Indicate how potential participants will be offered the option to take part in the study. Indicate who will request consent, what information they will convey, and how you will ensure each potential subject has sufficient time to make an informed decision about participating. Clarify how coercion and undue influence will be limited, particularly when recruiting from your patient population. If the study includes multiple sessions, describe how ongoing consent will be confirmed.

Write your consent form in lay terms at an approximate sixth to eighth grade reading level. Incorporate all required information including that the **study involves research**, is **voluntary**, and that **consent can be withdrawn**. List all **eligibility criteria, potential risks and benefits**, and investigator and IRB **contact information**. Include **signature lines** and indicate that **a copy will be given to each participant** (see **Appendix B**, Consent Form Requirements and Checklist, and Chapter 9).

If applicable, prepare copies of consent forms in more than one language. Include a copy of your consent form(s) with your IRB application materials.

Recruitment Methods

Explain how participants will be recruited and provide copies of any advertisements, including fliers or emails. Recruitment materials will include the **purpose** of the study, **eligibility** requirements, **activities** to be completed, **location** of the study, approximate **time commitment**, and **investigator** contact information (see **Appendix C**, Recruitment Methods and Checklist).

Medical Records

If applicable, explain who will access medical records, what information will be collected from the records, and whether any research-derived information will be added to the medical record.

Identifiable Data Collected

Indicate all participant identifiers that will be collected and describe how you will store and protect that information. Common identifiers include name, social security number, date of birth, medical record number, photos, images, and medical device serial numbers, among others. If you will de-identify data for analysis, indicate your procedures for doing so, describe how and where you will store the master list with identifying information, and indicate how and when that master list will be securely destroyed.

Data Safety and Monitoring

Describe plans, if any, to periodically monitor the data collected to evaluate harms and benefits. Describe any procedures for sharing data. Indicate how data will be collected and stored. Detail how confidentiality of the data will be maintained at all stages. Describe how electronic research data will be stored in a secured environment, using encrypted and password-protected devices, and where and how paper data will be shared and secured.

Conflicts of Interest

Each member of the study team must report any conflicts of interest (COI) to the IRB. COI are any activities or relationships that could compromise, or give the appearance of compromising, an investigator's ability to perform or report the research study. Examples include financial interests, such as consulting fees, stock options, or patents associated with materials in the study. Personal relationships and professional collaborations can also result in real or perceived conflicts of interest. Most institutions have COI forms detailing required disclosures. These forms are usually updated at least annually and any COI that arise during the study period are reported following your institution's procedures.

Attachments

Your IRB will indicate what information is required with your application. Common attachments include: the study **protocol** (narrative description of your study procedures), **consent forms**, **recruitment materials**, and all research materials including **surveys**, **questionnaires**, and **data collection tools** (e.g., spreadsheet).

Hint: Think about why the IRB needs the information asked for on the application. Remember, IRB members are not the enemy, and the committee does not exist to increase your workload. Reviewers simply need enough information to evaluate the purpose and procedures of the study and understand how participants will be protected from harm.

ALWAYS SUBMIT AMENDMENTS FOR ANY CHANGES TO AN APPROVED STUDY

Any changes you wish to make to an IRB approved study must first be submitted to the IRB for review. **All changes in research activity, including minor changes**, such as the addition or removal of study personnel or a data collection category, must be submitted to the IRB administrator **for evaluation prior to implementing the proposed changes**. This applies to studies that were approved through full committee, expedited, or exempt review processes.

Minor changes to studies previously approved through expedited or exempt review typically undergo expedited or administrative review, as appropriate. At times, changes to a previously exempt study move it from the exempt category to the expedited review category, and sometimes, though rare, to the full committee review category. Major changes to a research study previously approved through full committee review must be reviewed by the full committee.

8.5 APPRECIATE WHY PREPARING AN IRB APPLICATION IS HELPFUL

Before beginning your IRB application, it may be helpful to think about the benefits of the IRB preparation process. Granted, completing an application is usually the sort of task that seems more annoying than useful, and you will likely feel it is taking too much of your already limited time. However, the **IRB process** often **improves your research study and can end up saving you time in the long run**. Keeping these benefits in mind may help whenever you feel overburdened by the process (**Box 8.3**).

Why is writing an IRB application helpful? **The study details, materials, power analysis, statistical plans, recruitment, and consent procedures are explained in the IRB application**. These are all things you must do anyway. Thus, rather than wasting time, you are refining your study and creating materials that can be used in multiple contexts. Similar benefits arise when preparing an application for research involving animal models (**Box 8.4**).

Through preparing your IRB application materials:

1) **You create text that can be used for other documents**. Your IRB application and protocol include background information and previous findings that explain the need for your study. This is the **same information you include in the introduction** of a **manuscript** or **grant application**.

   The IRB application includes details of the **procedures** you will use. These procedures become the **Materials and Methods** section of a **manuscript** or **grant application**.

   You will likely have to revise and update portions of each section to fit the purpose of other documents, but the main work is done when you prepare your IRB application.

2) **You get feedback on study design**. The IRB is focused on protecting the participants. This includes **making sure the scientific design is appropriate for the question(s) asked** so subjects are not encountering risks for a project that will not result in meaningful data. Because the IRB reviews applications in this way, you often get helpful feedback that improves

your study. Early input can help **ensure** you have **data that is relevant and worth sharing**.

3) **You have all the materials needed to begin your study**. The IRB needs to see all the materials you are using. That may feel intrusive or outside the purview of the IRB, but it is neither. For example, the IRB needs to see your recruitment flier and consent forms to make sure you are recruiting fairly and appropriately and that you are providing all the information needed for potential subjects to make an informed decision. You also include your data collection tool and any survey questions or evaluations that you are planning to use. **Your materials are therefore reviewed by others** and **ready to use as soon as the IRB grants approval**.

4) **You know the number of participants needed for your study**. IRB applications require you to determine how many participants are needed for your study, usually with a power analysis. Without this calculation you risk having too few subjects for data analysis. As some investigators admit, they would skip the power analysis and simply make an educated guess about sample size if it was not required by the IRB. Thus, the IRB protects you from completing a study with an inadequate sample size.

Hint: Investigators unfamiliar with power analysis should consult a statistician for advice. A statistician may also assist in identifying any weaknesses in methodology that would limit the value of the study.

Box 8.3 Resident Perspective: Writing an IRB Application
Derek Damrow, M.D., Orthopaedic Surgery Resident

The IRB application may seem like a daunting task if it is the first time you have ever worked on one. Where do I begin? What do I need to include? Why is this even necessary? All these questions and more may come up and you are not the first, nor the last to have these feelings, though know that writing the IRB application may be the single most important part of your research. These are five of the things I would have liked to have known prior to starting my IRB application.

1. **Make a checklist**. Do this first, so you know whether you have all the relevant documents and information that you need. Every study is going to need to have a consent form (if working with human subjects) and protocol. Does your study require a questionnaire, survey, data collection log? These should all be added to your checklist.
2. **Be prepared**. This really is a continuation of the first point but is important, so it gets its own number. I cannot stress how important it is to be prepared. It all starts with your literature review. By performing an in-depth literature review, writing notes, compiling references, it will

help you not only to write your IRB application, but also this will be the backbone of the introduction for your manuscript. The more work you put in at the beginning, before you even attempt to start designing and getting the project started, the easier the final half will be.

3. **Be thorough**. What I mean by this is that, when writing the protocol, think of every little detail and every pitfall you may encounter, and how you are going to try to avoid or mitigate these problems. If you do not think of the potential pitfalls, the IRB committee will. That is part of their job in approving the study. If you can think of potential weaknesses, and address them prior to submitting the application to the IRB, this will help get the project approved. It also may prevent you from investing countless hours into a project only to find out your data are invalid or flawed due to a design error in your study that your research team and the IRB did not catch.

4. **Have open communication**. This may be an obvious point but is valuable. If you are designing the project, generating grants, and writing with a co-investigator, make sure you are telling each other what you are working on and sharing documents with one another. If you can, make a shared account that all members of the research team can access and place all documents that are worked on in that account. Many headaches will be had if one person does one part but wording or procedures are different from what you originally had planned, thus requiring alterations. Additionally, the IRB may request grant approval letters, grant applications, survey forms, etc. If you are not sharing with each other, it may delay your work and require multiple emails/texts/phone calls.

5. **Be patient**. You most likely will be asked to revise your study after your first submission. That is okay! No one nails it the first time. The IRB thinks of things that you may have overlooked or did not think of. This will save you in the long run. This may happen multiple times before your IRB application is finally approved. Once again, that is okay! Your study will be stronger because of it.

I hope these five points from a resident perspective help when it comes to writing your study protocol/IRB application. At the end of the day, it is a necessary part of research. Just be patient and flexible with it. Good luck!

Box 8.4: Research Involving Animal Models

Some research studies use animal models. As with clinical research involving human subjects, there are regulations to follow, training courses to complete, and applications to submit to an institutional committee before research begins.

Most institutions in the United States have an **Institutional Animal Care and Use Committee (IACUC)** that reviews applications for projects involving animal models. The IACUC is comprised of a minimum of five members including a veterinarian with expertise in laboratory animal care, a scientist with expertise working with animals in research, a non-scientist, and someone not associated with the institution. All IACUC members receive training and must update their credentials regularly. Like IRBs, most IACUCs include more than the minimum number of required members.

Applications undergo a full committee review or a designated member review, the latter being a form of expedited review. All applications are assessed to determine whether the **proposed use of animals is acceptable** and **appropriate** for the type of research being conducted. Investigators must justify their choice of species, indicate the number of animals they expect to use, and explain why other options (e.g., cell or tissue culture, computer simulation, another species) are not appropriate for the proposed research.

The committee considers these explanations as well as the planned housing and care of the animals throughout the study, planned experimental procedures, methods to address pain or distress, and forms of euthanasia. The IACUC evaluates the training of those involved in the work, the plans for veterinary care, and whether the work needlessly duplicates previous research.

For approved studies, the committee monitors the number of animals used and inspects the animal facilities at least twice per year. Investigators keep records of all animals used, including any that expire during the study period. The IACUC sends a report to the designated institutional official annually, detailing all animal research-related activities and any concerns.

In the United States, most institutions follow the same basic procedures. However, there are **different federal regulations** that depend, in part, on the **species used** and the **source of funding** for the research. Any investigator who works with live vertebrate animals and receives funding from a Public Health Services (PHS) agency (e.g., NIH, NSF) will follow the guidelines of the **Office of Laboratory Animal Welfare (OLAW)**. Funding is only awarded to an investigator if the institution has an approved animal welfare assurance on file.

Investigators who do not have PHS funding but receive other federal or private funding may follow the guidelines of the **United States Department of Agriculture Animal Welfare Act** (USDA AWA). USDA AWA does not cover rats, mice, or birds that are bred for research purposes. Thus, any research studies with these species are not governed by AWA policies.

Because researchers at any given institution could receive funding from federal or private agencies, many **institutions incorporate guidelines from all federal agencies to ensure all studies are compliant**. Thus, your institution may follow PHS policies even if no investigators have PHS funding and the only species used are mice bred for research purposes. Many institutions further demonstrate commitment to animal welfare by following guidelines of the international **Association for Assessment and Accreditation of Laboratory Animal Care** (AAALAC).

As a resident, you will work with senior members of your lab and your institution's IACUC to make sure you follow all required procedures. The resources at the end of this chapter will help you understand the different policies. You will also be required to complete training in appropriate care and use of animals through CITI or another mechanism at your institution.

Note: Invertebrate species are not covered by federal regulations though institutions may have procedures that must be followed.

Remember: Never begin any work with animals until you have received training and the study has been approved by the IACUC.

8.6 CONCLUSIONS

Any research study involving human subjects requires approval from the IRB to ensure participant rights are protected and investigators follow appropriate practices. Although many ethical guidelines appear to be common sense, it is surprisingly easy to overlook behaviors and practices that compromise participant rights, safety, or confidentiality.

Remember that the effort you put into developing a well-crafted IRB application is not wasted. You will have fewer revision requests from the IRB, leading to a faster approval process, as well as material that can be incorporated into future documents. If you ever find yourself frustrated with the IRB process and feel it is taking more time than necessary, remember you are saving time overall.

Keep in mind that the participants, who are often your patients, are volunteering their time and potentially exposing themselves to risks so you can collect data. Appreciate and respect their contribution to your work and take the time to develop a project that reflects your clinical standards and concern for your study participants.

APPENDIX A: CHARACTERISTICS OF STUDIES EVALUATED UNDER EXEMPT, EXPEDITED, AND FULL COMMITTEE REVIEW PROCEDURES

From the U.S. Department of Health and Human Services Office of Human Research Protections
   • **https://www.hhs.gov/ohrp/regulations-and-policy/regulations/45-cfr-46/index.html**

Note: Contact your IRB administrator for assistance in identifying the category of research and the application materials required by your institution. Check the OHRP website for any updates to the following:

EXEMPT RESEARCH

(Note: Investigators must receive written notification from the IRB that the study is exempt from IRB committee oversight prior to beginning the study.)

(1) Research, conducted in established or commonly accepted educational settings, that specifically involves normal educational practices that are not likely to adversely impact students' opportunity to learn required educational content or the assessment of educators who provide instruction. This includes most research on regular and special education instructional strategies, and research on the effectiveness of or the comparison among instructional techniques, curricula, or classroom management methods.

(2) Research that only includes interactions involving educational tests (cognitive, diagnostic, aptitude, achievement), survey procedures, interview procedures, or observation of public behavior (including visual or auditory recording) if at least one of the following criteria is met:

    (i) The information obtained is recorded by the investigator in such a manner that the identity of the human subjects cannot readily be ascertained, directly or through identifiers linked to the subjects;

    (ii) Any disclosure of the human subjects' responses outside the research would not reasonably place the subjects at risk of criminal or civil liability or be damaging to the subjects' financial standing, employability, educational advancement, or reputation; or

    (iii) The information obtained is recorded by the investigator in such a manner that the identity of the human subjects can readily be ascertained, directly or through identifiers linked to the subjects, and an IRB conducts a limited IRB review to make the determination required by §46.111(a)(7).

(3i) Research involving benign behavioral interventions in conjunction with the collection of information from an adult subject through verbal or written responses (including data entry) or audiovisual recording if the subject prospectively agrees to the intervention and information collection and at least one of the following criteria is met:

    (A) The information obtained is recorded by the investigator in such a manner that the identity of the human subjects cannot readily be ascertained, directly or through identifiers linked to the subjects;

    (B) Any disclosure of the human subjects' responses outside the research would not reasonably place the subjects at risk of criminal or civil liability or be damaging to the subjects' financial standing, employability, educational advancement, or reputation; or

    (C) The information obtained is recorded by the investigator in such a manner that the identity of the human subjects can readily be ascertained, directly or through identifiers linked to the subjects, and an IRB conducts a limited IRB review to make the determination required by §46.111(a)(7).

(ii) For the purpose of this provision, benign behavioral interventions are brief in duration, harmless, painless, not physically invasive, not likely to have a significant adverse lasting impact on the subjects, and the investigator has no reason to think the subjects will find the interventions offensive or embarrassing. Provided all such criteria are met, examples of such benign behavioral interventions would include having the subjects play an online game, having them solve puzzles under various noise conditions, or having them decide how to allocate a nominal amount of received cash between themselves and someone else.

(iii) If the research involves deceiving the subjects regarding the nature or purposes of the research, this exemption is not applicable unless the subject authorizes the deception through a prospective agreement to participate in research under circumstances in which the subject is informed that he or she will be unaware of or misled regarding the nature or purposes of the research.

(4) Secondary research for which consent is not required: secondary research uses of identifiable private information or identifiable biospecimens, if at least one of the following criteria is met:

(i)   The identifiable private information or identifiable biospecimens are publicly available;

(ii) Information, which may include information about biospecimens, is recorded by the investigator in such a manner that the identity of the human subjects cannot readily be ascertained directly or through identifiers linked to the subjects, the investigator does not contact the subjects, and the investigator will not re-identify subjects;

(iii) The research involves only information collection and analysis involving the investigator's use of identifiable health information when that use is regulated under 45 CFR parts 160 and 164, subparts A and E, for the purposes of "health care operations" or "research" as those terms are defined at 45 CFR 164.501 or for "public health activities and purposes" as described under 45 CFR 164.512(b); or

(iv) The research is conducted by, or on behalf of, a Federal department or agency using government-generated or government-collected information obtained for non-research activities, if the research generates identifiable private information that is or will be maintained on information technology that is subject to and in compliance with section 208(b) of the E-Government Act of 2002, 44 U.S.C. 3501 note, if all of the identifiable private information collected, used, or generated as part of the activity will be maintained in systems of records subject to the Privacy Act of 1974, 5 U.S.C. 552a, and, if applicable, the information used in the research was collected subject to the Paperwork Reduction Act of 1995, 44 U.S.C. 3501 *et seq.*

(5) Research and demonstration projects that are conducted or supported by a Federal department or agency, or are otherwise subject to

the approval of department or agency heads (or the approval of the heads of bureaus or other subordinate agencies that have been delegated authority to conduct the research and demonstration projects), and that are designed to study, evaluate, improve, or otherwise examine public benefit or service programs, including procedures for obtaining benefits or services under those programs, possible changes in or alternatives to those programs or procedures, or possible changes in methods or levels of payment for benefits or services under those programs. Such projects include, but are not limited to, internal studies by Federal employees, and studies under contracts or consulting arrangements, cooperative agreements, or grants. Exempt projects also include waivers of otherwise mandatory requirements using authorities such as sections 1115 and 1115A of the Social Security Act, as amended.

   (i)   Each Federal department or agency conducting or supporting the research and demonstration projects must establish, on a publicly accessible Federal Web site or in such other manner as the department or agency head may determine, a list of the research and demonstration projects that the Federal department or agency conducts or supports under this provision. The research or demonstration project must be published on this list prior to commencing the research involving human subjects.

(6) Taste and food quality evaluation and consumer acceptance studies:

   (i)   If wholesome foods without additives are consumed, or

   (ii)   If a food is consumed that contains a food ingredient at or below the level and for a use found to be safe, or agricultural chemical or environmental contaminant at or below the level found to be safe, by the Food and Drug Administration or approved by the Environmental Protection Agency or the Food Safety and Inspection Service of the U.S. Department of Agriculture.

(7) Storage or maintenance for secondary research for which broad consent is required: Storage or maintenance of identifiable private information or identifiable biospecimens for potential secondary research use if an IRB conducts a limited IRB review and makes the determinations required by §46.111(a)(8).

(8) Secondary research for which broad consent is required: Research involving the use of identifiable private information or identifiable biospecimens for secondary research use, if the following criteria are met:

   (i)   Broad consent for the storage, maintenance, and secondary research use of the identifiable private information or identifiable biospecimens was obtained in accordance with §46.116(a)(1) through (4), (a)(6), and (d);

   (ii)   Documentation of informed consent or waiver of documentation of consent was obtained in accordance with §46.117;

(iii)   An IRB conducts a limited IRB review and makes the determination required by §46.111(a)(7) and makes the determination that the research to be conducted is within the scope of the broad consent referenced in paragraph (d)(8)(i) of this section; and

(iv)   The investigator does not include returning individual research results to subjects as part of the study plan. This provision does not prevent an investigator from abiding by any legal requirements to return individual research results.

RESEARCH ELIGIBLE FOR EXPEDITED REVIEW

A.   Research activities that (1) present no more than minimal risk to human subjects, and (2) involve only procedures listed in one or more of the following categories, may be reviewed by the IRB through the expedited review procedure authorized by 45 CFR 46.110 and 21 CFR 56.110. The activities listed should not be deemed to be of minimal risk simply because they are included on this list. Inclusion on this list merely means that the activity is eligible for review through the expedited review procedure when the specific circumstances of the proposed research involve no more than minimal risk to human subjects.

B.   The categories in this list apply regardless of the age of subjects, except as noted.

C.   The expedited review procedure may not be used where identification of the subjects and/or their responses would reasonably place them at risk of criminal or civil liability or be damaging to the subjects' financial standing, employability, insurability, reputation, or be stigmatizing, unless reasonable and appropriate protections will be implemented so that risks related to invasion of privacy and breach of confidentiality are no greater than minimal.

D.   The expedited review procedure may not be used for classified research involving human subjects.

E.   IRBs are reminded that the standard requirements for informed consent (or its waiver, alteration, or exception) apply regardless of the type of review—expedited or convened—utilized by the IRB.

F.   Categories one (1) through seven (7) pertain to both initial and continuing IRB review.

Research Categories

1.   Clinical studies of drugs and medical devices only when condition (a) or (b) is met.

a.   Research on drugs for which an investigational new drug application (21 CFR Part 312) is not required. (Note: Research on marketed drugs that significantly increases the risks or decreases the acceptability of the risks associated with the use of the product is not eligible for expedited review.)

b. Research on medical devices for which (i) an investigational device exemption application (21 CFR Part 812) is not required; or (ii) the medical device is cleared/approved for marketing and the medical device is being used in accordance with its cleared/approved labeling.

2. Collection of blood samples by finger stick, heel stick, ear stick, or venipuncture as follows:

   a. from healthy, non-pregnant adults who weigh at least 110 pounds. For these subjects, the amounts drawn may not exceed 550 ml in an 8-week period and collection may not occur more frequently than two times per week; or

   b. from other adults and children, considering the age, weight, and health of the subjects, the collection procedure, the amount of blood to be collected, and the frequency with which it will be collected. For these subjects, the amount drawn may not exceed the lesser of 50 ml or 3 ml per kg in an 8-week period and collection may not occur more frequently than two times per week.

3. Prospective collection of biological specimens for research purposes by non-invasive means.

   Examples: (a) hair and nail clippings in a non-disfiguring manner; (b) deciduous teeth at time of exfoliation or if routine patient care indicates a need for extraction; (c) permanent teeth if routine patient care indicates a need for extraction; (d) excreta and external secretions (including sweat); (e) un-cannulated saliva collected either in an unstimulated fashion or stimulated by chewing gumbase or wax or by applying a dilute citric solution to the tongue; (f) placenta removed at delivery; (g) amniotic fluid obtained at the time of rupture of the membrane prior to or during labor; (h) supra- and subgingival dental plaque and calculus, provided the collection procedure is not more invasive than routine prophylactic scaling of the teeth and the process is accomplished in accordance with accepted prophylactic techniques; (i) mucosal and skin cells collected by buccal scraping or swab, skin swab, or mouth washings; (j) sputum collected after saline mist nebulization.

4. Collection of data through non-invasive procedures (not involving general anesthesia or sedation) routinely employed in clinical practice, excluding procedures involving X-rays or microwaves. Where medical devices are employed, they must be cleared/approved for marketing. (Studies intended to evaluate the safety and effectiveness of the medical device are not generally eligible for expedited review, including studies of cleared medical devices for new indications.)

   Examples: (a) physical sensors that are applied either to the surface of the body or at a distance and do not involve input of significant amounts of energy into the subject or an invasion of the subject's privacy; (b) weighing or testing sensory acuity; (c) magnetic resonance imaging; (d) electrocardiography, electroencephalography, thermography, detection of naturally occurring radioactivity, electroretinography, ultrasound, diagnostic infrared imaging, Doppler blood flow, and echocardiography; (e) moderate exercise, muscular strength testing, body composition assessment, and flexibility testing where appropriate, given the age, weight, and health of the individual.

5. Research involving materials (data, documents, records, or specimens) that have been collected, or will be collected solely for non-research purposes (such as medical treatment or diagnosis). (Note: Some research in this category may be exempt from the HHS regulations for the protection of human subjects. 45 CFR 46.101(b)(4). This listing refers only to research that is not exempt.)

6. Collection of data from voice, video, digital, or image recordings made for research purposes.

7. Research on individual or group characteristics or behavior (including, but not limited to, research on perception, cognition, motivation, identity, language, communication, cultural beliefs or practices, and social behavior) or research employing survey, interview, oral history, focus group, program evaluation, human factor evaluation, or quality assurance methodologies. (Note: some research in this category may be exempt from the HHS regulations for the protection of human subjects. 45 CFR 46.101(b)(2) and (b)(3). This listing refers only to research that is not exempt.)

8. Continuing review of research previously approved by the convened IRB as follows:
   a. where (i) the research is permanently closed to the enrollment of new subjects; (ii) all subjects have completed all research-related interventions; and (iii) the research remains active only for long-term follow-up of subjects; or
   b. where no subjects have been enrolled and no additional risks have been identified; or
   c. where the remaining research activities are limited to data analysis.

9. Continuing review of research, not conducted under an investigational new drug application or investigational device exemption where categories two (2) through eight (8) do not apply but the IRB has determined and documented at a convened meeting that the research involves no greater than minimal risk and no additional risks have been identified.

RESEARCH REQUIRING FULL COMMITTEE REVIEW

All studies that involve risk of physical or psychological harm greater than that encountered in daily life or during routine examinations or tests.

An IRB may also require full committee review for studies of any level of risk if the study involves vulnerable populations, sensitive topics, genetic testing, or a complex research design that requires expertise from multiple IRB members to effectively evaluate.

APPENDIX B: ELEMENTS OF INFORMED CONSENT

The consent form is an extremely important piece of the IRB application. The consent form provides participants with all the information they need to make an informed decision about whether to participate in the study. The form is also a reminder for all who work with the participants to adhere to the contract of the consent form (see also Chapter 9).

The consent form is written in a manner accessible to participants of all ages and backgrounds.

Some IRB members review the consent form before any other part of the application. If they cannot understand the project and the role of the participant, then it is unlikely potential participants will either.

Nine Basic Elements Required in All Consent Forms

1. A statement that the study involves research, an explanation of the purposes of the research, the expected duration of the subject's participation, a description of the procedures to be followed, and identification of any procedures that are experimental
2. A description of any reasonably foreseeable risks or discomforts to the subject
3. A description of any benefits to the subject or to others that may reasonably be expected from the research.
4. A disclosure of appropriate alternative procedures or courses of treatment, if any, that might be advantageous to the subject
5. A statement describing the extent, if any, to which confidentiality of records identifying the subject will be maintained
6. For research involving more than minimal risk, an explanation as to whether any compensation and an explanation as to whether any medical treatments are available if injury occurs, and, if so, what they consist of, or where further information may be obtained
7. An explanation of whom to contact for answers to pertinent questions about the research and research subjects' rights, and whom to contact in the event of a research-related injury to the subject
8. A statement that participation is voluntary, refusal to participate will involve no penalty or loss of benefits to which the subject is otherwise entitled, and the subject may discontinue participation at any time without penalty or loss of benefits to which the subject is otherwise entitled
9. One of the following statements about any research that involves the collection of identifiable private information or identifiable biospecimens:

A.   A statement that identifiers might be removed from the identifiable private information or identifiable biospecimens and that, after such removal, the information or biospecimens could be used for future research studies or distributed to another investigator for future research studies without additional informed consent from the subject or the legally authorized representative, if this might be a possibility **OR**

B.   A statement that the subject's information or biospecimens collected as part of the research, even if identifiers are removed, will not be used or distributed for future research studies.

Nine Additional Elements of Informed Consent to Be Included Where Appropriate

1.   A statement that the particular treatment or procedure may involve risks to the subject (or embryo or fetus, if the subject is or may become pregnant) that are currently unforeseeable

2.   Anticipated circumstances under which the subject's participation may be terminated by the investigator without regard to the subject's or the legally authorized representative's consent

3.   Any additional costs to the subject that may result from participation in the research

4.   The consequences of a subject's decision to withdraw from the research and procedures for orderly termination of participation by the subject

5.   A statement that significant new findings developed during the course of the research that may relate to the subject's willingness to continue participation will be provided to the subject

6.   The approximate number of subjects involved in the study

7.   A statement that the subject's biospecimens (even if identifiers are removed) may be used for commercial profit and whether the subject will or will not share in this commercial profit

8.   A statement regarding whether clinically relevant research results, including individual research results, will be disclosed to subjects, and if so, under what conditions

9.   For research involving biospecimens, whether the research will (if known) or might include whole-genome sequencing (i.e., sequencing of a human germline or somatic specimen with the intent to generate the genome or exome sequence of that specimen)

APPENDIX C: RECRUITMENT MATERIALS

Investigators must think about where and how participants will be recruited and how to avoid bias in recruitment practices. The IRB evaluates whether investigators select participants in a fair and ethical manner and refrain from coercing or discouraging participation for any reason.

Recruitment materials are written in lay language easily understood by the target population and include:

1. Name and address of the investigator and or research facility/institution
2. Purpose of research
3. Inclusion/exclusion criteria
4. Brief list of procedures involved
5. Time or other commitment required (number of visits, total duration including follow-up visits, etc.)
6. Location of research and contact person for further information

REFERENCES AND RESOURCES FOR HUMAN SUBJECTS RESEARCH

BOOKS
Levine, Robert J. *Ethics and Regulation of Clinical Research.* Baltimore, MD: Urban and Schwarzenberg; 1981.

REPORTS

THE NUREMBERG CODE
- https://history.nih.gov/display/ history/Nuremberg+Code

DECLARATION OF GENEVA (2006 VERSION)
- https:// www.wma.net/wp-content/uploads/2018/07/Decl-of-Geneva-v2006-1.pdf

WORLD MEDICAL ASSOCIATION DECLARATION OF HELSINKI
- https://jamanetwork.com/journals/jama/fullarticle/1760318

THE BELMONT REPORT
National Commission for the Protection of Human Subjects of Biomedical and Behavioral Research, *The Belmont Report, 1979.*
- https://www.hhs.gov/ohrp/regulations-and-policy/belmont-report/index.html

ONLINE TRAINING FOR PROTECTION OF HUMAN SUBJECTS
U.S. Health and Human Services (HHS) Office for Human Research Protections (OHRP) offers online training modules for investigators, key personnel, and IRB members. Access is free and viewers can print a certificate upon completing each of the four lessons.
- www.hhs.gov/ohrp/education-and-outreach/online-education/human-research-protection-training/index.html

REFERENCES AND RESOURCES FOR RESEARCH WITH ANIMAL MODELS

IACUC
- https://olaw.nih.gov/resources/tutorial/iacuc.htm

PHS Policy on Humane Care and Use of Laboratory Animals
- https://olaw.nih.gov/policies-laws/phs-policy.htm

Guide for the Care and Use of Laboratory Animals: 8th edition
- https://www.nap.edu/catalog/12910/gide-for/the-care-and-use-of-laboratory-animals-eighth

USDA APHIS
- https://www.aphis.usda.gov/aphis/ourfocus/animalwelfare/sa_awa

Animal Research Regulations in the U.S.—Speaking of Research
- https://speakingofresearch.com/facts/research-regulation

Obtaining Informed Consent for Research Studies

Lynne M. Bianchi, Ph.D.

Tips for Success:

> Practice your informed consent procedures before meeting with potential participants.
> Rehearse how you will respond to likely questions and concerns.

Warning:

> Consent discussions and your responsibilities to participants do not end when the consent form is signed.

Key Concept: The informed consent process involves ongoing conversation between members of the research team and study participants.

Clinical studies with human subjects typically require informed consent. The concept of informed consent is as simple as it sounds. **Individuals agree to participate in a study based on an accurate understanding of what the study involves**; their decision is fully informed.

As explained in Chapter 8, part of the informed consent process involves giving participants a copy of the **consent form** approved by your Institutional Review Board (IRB). However, informed consent is much more than sharing a form. It includes the initial discussion inviting participation and ongoing conversations throughout the study. During these conversations, you may provide additional information or address participant concerns. With every conversation, you ascertain whether an enrolled participant wishes to continue in the study.

The informed consent **document** and **discussions** focus on conveying information in a manner **comprehensible** to the individual being asked to participate in the study. Informed consent is not possible if an individual misunderstands the voluntary nature of participation or cannot follow study procedures due to a language barrier or cognitive impairment. As an investigator, **you are responsible for ensuring all participants are fully informed prior to enrolling**.

DOI: 10.1201/9781003126478-9

This chapter describes how to communicate the information included in your IRB-approved consent form in an effective and appropriate manner to optimize comprehension and minimize undue influence and coercion. Effective communication involves more than simply reading the form to someone. Therefore, you must practice what you will say and prepare how you will address questions and concerns that arise.

Many of the examples in this chapter relate to patients enrolling in a clinical research study. However, the elements of informed consent apply to all studies and all participants, including projects that recruit students or colleagues.

Remember: As an investigator, you need to be adept at communicating the elements of informed consent. You must explain the information in your consent form in a non-threatening, non-coercive manner that encourages questions from the individual you are asking to be in the study.

Note: If specific criteria are met, your Institutional Review Board (IRB) or ethics committee may grant a waiver of informed consent or a waiver of informed consent documentation (**Box 9.1**). For example, waivers may be given for studies of de-identified private information or de-identified biospecimens that do not present more than minimal risk to participants. Investigators must justify the need for such waivers or alterations and explain why the research could not be practicably carried out without the waiver or alteration. Such requests must be reviewed and approved by the committee before investigators begin any study.

Box 9.1   Waiver or Alterations of Informed Consent

Under specific circumstances, the informed consent procedures described in this chapter may not be required. **Any waiver or alteration to the informed consent process must meet specific federal criteria** and be **approved by the IRB** or ethics committee prior to initiating the study.

Waivers or alterations of consent procedures may be considered if:

1) the research is to be conducted by or subject to the approval of state or local government officials and is designed to study, evaluate, or otherwise examine one of the following:

a. public benefit or service programs
b. procedures for obtaining benefits or services under those programs
c. possible changes in or alternatives to those programs or procedures
d. possible changes in methods or levels of payment for benefits or services under those programs; *or*

2) The research involves no more than minimal risk to the subjects; *and*
3) the research could not practicably be carried out without the waiver or alteration.

9.1 PRESENT THE ELEMENTS OF INFORMED CONSENT EFFECTIVELY

Informed consent requires that potential participants are given the **required information** and **sufficient time** to decide whether they wish to join a study. The informed consent document and conversations include discussion of the **voluntary** nature of participation, the study **purpose, methods, duration, risks, benefits, confidentiality** of records, **contact** information for questions or concerns, and, if applicable, alternative **approaches, compensation, costs to participants**, and protocols for **study-related injury**.

As an investigator, you must consider and prepare for the many scenarios that interfere with an informed consent. For example, when your study population includes those whose primary language is not English, consent forms will be provided in more than one language. If necessary, you will arrange for a translator to be present during the initial conversation and all follow-up conversations.

Always remain cognizant of potential misunderstandings and consider how individual circumstances can influence comprehension and decision making. A person arriving to the emergency room may not be able to process the information clearly because they are injured or scared. Someone with a serious medical condition might misunderstand the risks of participating because they are so desperate for a potential cure.

UNDERSTAND RECENT REVISIONS TO INFORMED CONSENT PROCEDURES

In **January 2019**, changes were made to the United States Code of Federal Regulations (the "**Common Rule**") to address ongoing concerns about existing consent procedures. The **revised** requirements for informed consent include **nine basic elements** and **nine additional elements** (see checklist in Chapter 8, Appendix B). Most of these elements were already in practice; only one new basic element and three new additional elements were added.

The revised Common Rule, also called the **Final Rule**, was initiated to improve document content, reduce investigator and IRB administrative tasks, and address scientific advances (e.g., whole-genome sequencing).

One motivation for revising the Common Rule was growing concern about the way information was presented in consent documents. In some cases, consent forms appeared to entice participation rather than provide a neutral, informative overview of the study. Other consent forms read like legal documents, protecting investigators and institutions from liability. Many were simply too long, with key information scattered throughout the document. Lengthy and disorganized presentations make it unnecessarily difficult to process the content and make an informed decision about enrolling.

To focus the consent process on participant comprehension, the **updated regulations** require: (1) **organization** and **explanations** that **aid decision making**;

(2) **key information** presented **early in the document**; and (3) content written from "**a reasonable person perspective**." That is, documents containing the information most people need to make an informed decision.

Key elements included at the beginning of most consent documents are listed in **A–D below**. Other elements (E-N) are often included later in the document. However, because the focus is on organizing the document in a logical manner that aids comprehension, the final order may differ for any given study.

Note: Investigators of any clinical trial supported by a U.S. federal department or agency are now required to post a copy of the IRB-approved consent form on the clincaltrials.gov website.

PRESENT THE CONSENT DOCUMENT ACCURATELY, EFFECTIVELY, AND ETHICALLY

Study team members who invite potential participants to join a study often begin by emphasizing the voluntary nature of participation and give a brief overview of the study purpose before reviewing the entire consent document. For example, "We are enrolling volunteers in a research study to test a new medical device that measures glucose in people with type I diabetes. I will describe the study to you, but please note you are not required to volunteer, and your medical care will not change if you decide not to be in the study."

Each item in the consent form is then discussed, being careful not to omit, revise, or misrepresent the information contained in the document.

Note: Practice your consent conversation with a research team member or other colleague to get feedback. Address areas in need of improvement before you meet with any potential participants.

Tip: Write a script to follow to ensure that you provide the same information each time.

Hint: Anticipate questions you may be asked and develop appropriate answers to them.

Each time you go through the consent document, **pause to invite questions and comments**. Some areas of the consent form may require special attention, as illustrated in the examples below.

Research Purpose and Procedures

One of the first points to explain to potential participants is that you are asking them to participate in a research study. Many patients are unfamiliar with clinical research practices so **confirm that the person understands how a research study differs from standard medical care.**

Next, explain the **purpose** of the study, the **procedures** involved, and the **time commitment** required of participants. If any of the procedures are experimental, that must be emphasized. If participants are assigned to **groups**, explain how that is done and indicate whether the person can select or change groups. This introduction to the study purpose and methods should **clarify what is expected of those who choose to enroll**.

The World Health Organization Research Ethics Review Committee (WHO ERC) provides the following examples in their informed consent form template for clinical studies.

Study Purpose: *Malaria is one of the most common and dangerous diseases in this region. The drugs that are currently used to help people with malaria are not as good as we would like them to be. In fact, only 40 out of every 100 people given the malaria drug XYZ are completely cured. There is a new drug which may work better. The reason we are doing this research is to find out if the new drug ABX is better than drug XYZ which is currently being used.*

Time Commitment: *The research takes place over ___ (number of) days/or ___ (number of) months in total. During that time, it will be necessary for you to come to the clinic/hospital/health facility for _____(number of) days, for ____ (number of) hours each day. We would like to meet with you three months after your last clinic visit for a final check-up.*

In total, you will be asked to come 5 times to the clinic in 6 months. At the end of 6 months, the research will be finished.

Group assignment: *Because we do not know if the new malaria drug is better than the currently available drug for treating malaria, we need to compare the two. To do this, we will put people taking part in this research into two groups. The groups are selected by chance, as if by tossing a coin.*

Participants in one group will be given the test drug while participants in the other group will be given the drug that is currently being used for malaria. It is important that neither you nor we know which of the two drugs you are given. This information will be in our files, but we will not look at these files until after the research is finished. This is the best way we have for testing without being influenced by what we think or hope might happen. We will then compare which of the two has the best results.

Procedures: *This research will involve a single injection in your arm as well as four follow-up visits to the clinic.*

In the first visit, a small amount of blood, equal to about a teaspoon, will be taken from your arm with a syringe. This blood will be tested for the presence of substances that help your body to fight infections. We will also ask you a few questions about your general health and measure how tall you are and how much you weigh.

At the next visit, which will be 2 weeks later, you will again be asked some questions about your health and then you will be given either the test drug or the drug that is currently used for malaria. As explained before, neither you nor we will know whether you have received the test or the dummy/pretend drug.

After 1 week, you will come back to the clinic for a blood test. This will involve....

Changing groups: *The health care workers will be looking after you and the other participants very carefully during the study. If we are concerned about what the drug is doing, we will find out which drug you are getting and make changes. If there is anything you are concerned about or that is bothering you about the research, please talk to me or one of the other researchers.*

Voluntary Participation and the Right to Withdraw at Any Time with No Penalty or Loss of Benefits

For patients, benefits are often thought of in terms of medical care. Patients need to be reassured that their medical care will not be altered based their enrollment or withdrawal status.

Patients also need to understand that they do not need to "help" you and that you will not be upset if they decline. Be careful not to appear pleased or disappointed by a patient's decision.

When you explain that the participant can withdraw at any time, be careful not to imply the patient should go ahead and enroll, then decide later whether they will participate.

Remember: At any point during the consent process a person may decide not to participate. Some will tell you why they are not interested, others will decline without explanation. In either case, you accept the decision, thank the person for considering study participation, and end the consent discussion.

Potential Risks and Discomforts

Risks may include potential serious medical complications, side effects such as dizziness, or discomforts such as temporary muscle soreness. **All risks** and **discomforts** are **explained** in a neutral manner without downplaying or overstressing any risk. Procedures to minimize or treat any adverse effects are also described.

In some studies, specific types of risks may need to be addressed such as:

> *Unforeseen risks.* In some cases, the severity of risks will not be known, such as when a new medication or treatment is being tested. Explain the possibility of unknown risks and why they

are unknown. Be prepared to answer questions about the likelihood and nature of unforeseen risks. Confirm that the person understands there could be short- or long-term effects that no one knows about.

Risks associated with withdrawing from the study. Participants can withdraw at any time, but they must be informed if stopping abruptly would pose a health risk. For example, a medication may need to be tapered off or a follow-up exam may be needed to safely withdraw from a study.

The necessary procedures to withdraw safely must be included in the consent document so participants have a record of that information. Confirm that participants understand the procedures to follow should they choose to leave the study.

Risk to loss of confidentiality. For most studies, there is a risk to confidentiality. You will explain how all medical information and study data will be collected and stored and indicate who will have access to that information. You will describe your procedures for protecting confidentiality. However, you must also clarify that it is possible, even if unlikely, that the information may be seen by someone else. If known, give examples of the types of individuals who might see their information.

There are many reasons participants may not wish to risk having their data or personal information seen by others. Some may consider the information collected too personal to risk having it exposed. For some, it may be acceptable to risk having another health care professional see the data but not someone outside the medical field, such as a university research collaborator.

Note: All consent processes, even those for minimal-risk studies, must describe how confidentiality of identifying information will be protected.

Benefits

Any expected advantages *directly* related to study participation are listed as benefits. For example, an educational intervention or therapeutic treatment included as part of the study design may offer potential benefits to those who enroll.

Including *indirect* benefits, such as additional doctor visits, is usually optional. Check with your IRB for preferred practices regarding indirect benefits. If included, clarify that the indirect benefits are not due to the study itself and, if applicable, explain how the same benefits could be obtained without participating in the study.

For many studies, there are no known direct benefits. A statement indicating there are no known benefits to participating in the study is included in the consent form and discussion.

Unless required by your IRB, there is no need to explain that data gathered may benefit scientific knowledge or future patients. If such a statement is included, it must be emphasized that the value of potential future benefits is unknown.

Tip: It is important not to "oversell" any benefits or make it appear that participants have an advantage over those not enrolled in the study.

Hint: Participating in research is not a benefit, nor is the feeling of satisfaction one may have for contributing to a research study.

Contact Information

The consent form includes the names, phone numbers, and email addresses of individuals to contact with any questions or concerns about study procedures, participants' rights, or research-related injuries. **Contact information for the investigators and the IRB is always included in this section**. Additional contacts are added based on the nature of the study.

Remind the participants to keep the contact information in an easily accessed location should they need to contact any study personnel.

This section may be included at the end of the document where it is easy to find, or a separate contact form may be provided. Easy access is especially important when adverse events are possible.

Note: The contact information needs to be complete, and any phone number or email address listed must be monitored regularly, and, if necessary, 24 hours a day.

Alternative Procedures

If there are relevant procedures or treatments besides those used in the study, those need to be covered during the consent process. For example, if an established standard of care is known to benefit the patient's condition, that must be described.

Again, the emphasis is on providing information and giving the person time to decide whether to participate. Each person will have a different perspective on the value of participating *versus* pursuing other options; your role is to provide the information needed to make an informed decision.

Compensation and Incentives

For some studies, participants may receive some form of compensation, such as reimbursement for gas mileage or a small stipend. As noted in Chapter 8, compensation must be reasonable and related to the requirements of participation. Incentives such as gift cards or being entered in a raffle may be offered for some studies. If a raffle is used, you must explain how the winner will be selected, when the prize will be awarded, and the approximate odds of winning.

The consent form and your conversation must also detail what happens to any compensation or incentive should a participant withdraw. Some incentives are given even if a participant withdraws before completing the study. For example, if a $10 gift card is offered for participating in an online survey or a 1-hour behavioral assessment, the gift card is given even if the participant answers only one survey question or stops the behavioral assessment after 15 minutes. The voluntary nature of participation and the right to withdraw must be maintained.

If a longer-term study involves multiple sessions, participants may receive the compensation or incentive for the sessions attended prior to withdrawal. This must be stated in the consent form and explained during the consent process.

As you review the consent document, check that the individual understands the criteria for receiving any compensation or incentive. Be careful not to make the compensation or incentive sound so appealing that it influences the decision to participate. You need to be certain participants do not consent simply to receive what is offered.

Tip: If your study includes a raffle prize, confirm participants understand they are not being given that prize.

Hint: Compensation and incentives are not benefits and cannot be presented as such.

Compensation for Research-Related Injury

When applicable, the consent process must explain the possibility that the research protocol could injure participants. The consent form and your discussion must explain what medical treatments and compensation will be provided in the event of a research-related injury. If the costs associated with any research-related injury will *not* be covered, that must be clearly stated. Contact information for those who will address any research-related injuries is also included, as noted above.

For example, your informed consent form may state, "It is possible that you could develop injuries (list likely injuries) from participating in this research study. In the event of injury resulting from this research, medical treatment is available but will be provided at the usual charge. It is the policy of this institution to provide neither financial compensation nor free medical treatment for a research-related injury."

Alternatively, if the institution or study sponsor will provide compensation, your informed consent document might state, "If injuries occur that are the result of participation in this study, (name of reimbursing party) will reimburse the standard charges for the treatment of these injuries. The compensation described in this section will be the only form of compensation provided to you for complications or injuries related to this study."

For studies where the risk of an injury is likely, it is important to rehearse how you will present this section. You will need to present the information in a matter-of-fact manner, be prepared to answer questions that arise, and have information available for any additional resources or contacts helpful to participants.

Exculpatory Language Is Not Permitted

Any language that appears to release the investigators, their institutions, or sponsors from blame is unacceptable. The consent document must not imply that the participant waives legal rights and cannot suggest or appear to suggest that investigators or institutions are free from any fault, guilt, negligence, or malpractice. Further, the consent document cannot release or appear to release the investigator, sponsor, or institution from liability for negligence.

An example from the U.S. FDA (2014) provides a comparison of acceptable and unacceptable ways to present a study.

1) *Acceptable*: In the event you suffer a research-related injury, your medical expenses will be your responsibility or that of your third-party payer, although you are not precluded from seeking to collect compensation for injury related to malpractice, fault, or blame on the part of those involved in the research.

2) *Unacceptable*: In the event you suffer a research-related injury, your medical expenses will be your responsibility or that of your third-party payer.

The IRB will review your consent form to ensure you include the correct language. When presenting the consent document, **use only the approved language** and confirm that participants understand they have rights that do not change upon entering the study.

Hint: As with the description of potential research-related injuries, this section can feel uncomfortable to explain. Rehearse your presentation and your answers to likely questions. Be prepared to refer the participant to other resources, if needed.

Additional Costs from Participating

In some cases, participants incur expenses for participating in a study. Any potential costs must be explained during the consent process. For example, if a participant or his insurance company will be charged for exams, tests, or treatments related to the study, those must be detailed in the consent document and explained during the consent discussion.

In some instances, an insurance company will not cover the costs for services associated with a research study. This too would need to be explained. If necessary, you can refer potential participants to a financial counselor or reimbursement specialist at your institution. This would be done prior to the patient signing the consent form.

Additionally, if a participant is likely to lose time from work or incur expenses related to travel to a research site, those too must be addressed in the consent form and discussion. Clarify if such costs are likely to exceed the amount of any compensation or reimbursement offered.

Note: Be prepared to refer individuals to the appropriate resources and personnel for information on any possible financial burdens associated with participation in the study.

Remember: Do not accept a signed consent form until you are certain that the participant understands the potential expenses that may be incurred.

Withdrawing from the Study

At times, an investigator may withdraw a participant from the study. For example**, investigator-initiated withdrawal** may occur if the participant does not follow the research protocol or misses required follow-up sessions. The criteria for investigator-initiated withdrawal are detailed in the consent form and, if withdrawal becomes necessary, **participants are informed why they were withdrawn**.

Note that **participant-initiated withdrawal** may occur at any time, but the **participant does not have to give a reason for choosing to leave the study**.

Whether investigator- or participant-initiated withdrawal, if there are treatments, protocols, or follow-up appointments required to **protect the well-being of the participant upon study withdrawal**, those are explained in the consent form and reviewed during informed consent conversations.

Make sure all participants are clear on how to safely withdraw from the study. Participants may need periodic reminders during the study, so they do not jeopardize their health by leaving the study without following established protocols.

The consent process also explains what, if any, **data** collected prior to withdrawal can be **excluded from analysis**. If there are conditions that impact when data can be withdrawn, those are explained. For example, if the data are de-identified and the master list has been destroyed before a participant withdraws, it would not be possible to identify that participant's data for exclusion. If data were already presented at a conference or appeared in a publication prior to withdrawal, the participant's data could no longer be excluded.

Note: Many participants will not be familiar with conference presentations, medical publication procedures, or methods of data analysis. Therefore, you need to discuss these issues in a manner that makes it clear what happens to the information you collect and when participant data can and cannot be excluded.

Number of Subjects

The number of subjects the study plans to enroll provides information that may sway the decision of some participants. Is your study a small, preliminary study or part of a larger, clinical trial? Some individuals may be more inclined to participate in one or the other. Although this recommended element of informed consent is not required under the revised Common Rule, your IRB may request this information as it aids decision making.

Biospecimens and Identifiable Personal Information

The Revised Common Rule added one basic element and two additional elements related to identifiable biospecimens and personal information. Mechanisms for broad consent for use of these materials were also added (**Box 9.2**):

1) All studies that acquire **identifiable biospecimens** (e.g., blood samples, tissue biopsy, buccal swab, amniotic fluid) or **identifiable private information** (e.g., name, date of birth, medical record number) must include one of the following:
   a. A statement that identifiers might be removed from the identifiable private information or identifiable biospecimens and that, after such removal, the information or biospecimens could be used for future research studies or distributed to another investigator for future research studies without additional informed consent from the subject or the legally authorized representative, if this might be a possibility; or
   b. A statement that the subject's information or biospecimens collected as part of the research, even if identifiers are removed, will *not* be used or distributed for future research studies.

If you include the second statement to indicate information or biospecimens will *not* be used in the future, then you and your study team are obligated to abide by that statement. Therefore, if there is any possibility that you may use participant information in the future, it is usually best to include statement (a). If you are unsure which to use, consult your IRB.

Tip: When known, explain the purpose of using the de-identified data in future studies.

Hint: Be prepared to explain the difference between identifiable and de-identified information. Although seemingly self-evident, many participants are unfamiliar with the procedures and purposes of de-identifying information.

2) When relevant, two additional elements of informed consent related to biospecimens are included:
   a. A statement that the subject's biospecimens (even if identifiers are removed) may be used for **commercial profit** and whether the participant will or will not share in this commercial profit.

   This may seem like an unlikely possibility but some biospecimens could lead to the generation of a cell line or reagents that are later sold to other investigators. If there are no plans for compensation, simply state "Biospecimens obtained from you in this research may help in the development of a commercial product. There are no plans to provide financial compensation to you should this occur."

   You may need to explain this section in more detail, so have a clear explanation of what types of products might be developed, who would develop them, and what portion of the biospecimen would be likely be used in developing such a product. Be clear whether this is a planned activity or a possible future use of biospecimens acquired during the study.
   b. A statement indicating whether the research will or might include **whole-genome sequencing** (sequencing with the intent to generate the genome or exome sequence of that specimen).

   You will explain what whole-genome sequencing means, how the information will be used in your study, and whether any information will be shared with the participants. If you plan to share information, you must also explain the potential impact of such information on participants and their family members. If applicable, resources such as genetic counselors or other health care providers are listed.

Hint: Be prepared to clarify what information is and is not obtained from whole-genome sequencing.

Box 9.2   Broad Consent

The Revised Common Rule provides an option to use a broad consent mechanism in which **participants grant permission to use their identifiable biospecimens or identifiable private information in future studies**. Broad consent can be incorporated into an existing informed consent document or can be sought for individual studies.

Broad consent documents include a description of the types of research likely to use the identifiable private information or biospecimens and a statement that consent is voluntary. Participants are told about any data sharing that may occur, the institutions or researchers who may work with their data, the period the data will be stored and used, and any foreseeable risks or benefits. The methods for maintaining confidentiality are also described. When applicable, the broad consent document discusses potential commercial profits, whole-genome sequencing, and whether results will be shared with participants. All necessary contact information is provided.

Broad consent requires tracking to ensure information or biospecimens are only accessed for those who have consented and that no information or biospecimens are used from those who declined or withdrew consent. Due to the complexity of such tracking, not all institutions have adopted broad consent. Check with your IRB for their current policies.

The **earlier procedures** for obtaining consent to use personal information or biospecimens in future studies **remain in place**. Thus, an investigator can request a waiver of informed consent from the IRB to work with de-identified biospecimens or de-identified private information. Alternatively, participants can be asked for consent to use their identifiable materials or information for a specific study.

Note: A waiver for consent cannot be granted for an individual who declined to give broad consent.

Disclosure of Clinically Relevant Results

The third new additional element addresses sharing clinically relevant findings, including individual research results, with participants. If results are to be shared, the consent form indicates how and when that will occur. If results will not be shared, that is stated.

Because there are benefits and risks to sharing information with participants, the IRB will assess whether the benefits of disclosing the information outweigh any potential risks. For example, sharing information may be appropriate if the information was gathered as part of standard-of-care and disclosing information has the potential to benefit the participant's health. However, if the data obtained would not impact health care, there may be no benefit in sharing the information. In other cases, it may not be possible to share information because the data were de-identified prior to analysis.

If any shared results are potentially distressing, resources for those who can assist participants in interpreting and processing the findings should be provided.

Note: Every member of the research team, whether involved in the initial consent process or not, should be familiar with the consent document and be able to direct participants to the proper resources whenever questions or concerns arise.

9.2 MINIMIZE COERCION AND UNDUE INFLUENCE

Whenever you or a member of your research team present an informed consent document or answer participant questions, it is essential that the conversations be free of coercion and undue influence. **Coercion** refers to intimidation or a threat of harm. **Undue influence** means a person is swayed to do something, often without considering the consequences.

CONSIDER HOW OTHERS PERCEIVE YOUR REQUEST TO PARTICIPATE IN A RESEARCH STUDY

You do not have to say or do anything out of the ordinary for others to feel coerced or unduly influenced to participate in your research study. Some of your patients will feel intimidated simply because you are a physician. Some may agree to participate because they are concerned you will not provide the same level of care if they decline. Others may consent because they want to please you. Junior colleagues or students may feel compelled to consent to avoid a negative evaluation.

Because of the many possible reactions from potential participants, you need to develop consent procedures that minimize perceptions of coercion and undue influence. One way to minimize such perceptions is to provide potential participants with **sufficient time to make an informed decision**. An investigator presenting a study to a patient an hour before surgery is not providing adequate time for the patient to ask questions or consider whether it is in his best interest to enroll.

It is also important to think about who presents the consent document and where consent conversations take place. In some cases, it may be best if the patient's physician does not initiate the consent process. Another member of the research team might discuss the consent document, with the physician available to address questions and concerns.

Whoever leads the consent discussions, **conversations must take place in a private location.** This prevents personal information from being overheard by others and encourages questions and concerns to be expressed.

UNDERSTAND VULNERABILITIES OF MARGINALIZED GROUPS

In addition to identified vulnerable populations (pregnant women, children, prisoners, cognitively impaired individuals), you are likely to discuss your study with members of various marginalized groups. Marginalization may stem from one's level of education, socio-economic status, disability status, race, ethnicity, gender, sexual orientation, or any other defining characteristic. Some individuals in these groups may be especially susceptible to feelings of coercion and undue influence. As with all consent and assent (**Box 9.3**) conversations, pay attention to how an individual reacts to your presentation and, if necessary, adapt your approach to encourage dialogue and questions.

Note, however, that, even as you encourage questions, many people will feel uncomfortable asking them. Some may feel it is disrespectful, some may feel they do not know enough about the topic to question the study. Some may feel too nervous or intimidated. It may be helpful to offer questions others have asked to help stimulate conversation. For example, "Some people have asked me how painful the injection might be, and some have wanted to know more about what happens when they come to the clinic for the first visit, have you been wondering about anything like that?"

Note that others may have unrealistic expectations that need to be addressed. For example, individuals with a chronic medical condition may feel compelled to join a study to receive an experimental treatment, without understanding they may be assigned to the placebo group. Others may overlook the possibility that side effects of the treatment could impact their quality of life. Make sure that all potential participants comprehend that they are enrolling in a research study, not a treatment program. When needed, review the procedures for group assignment and side effects.

Remember: As an investigator, you want to enroll as many eligible individuals as possible in your study. However, you must do so in a manner that ensures those who enroll do so in a fully informed manner and not in response to any feelings of coercion or undue influence.

Box 9.3   Understand the Difference between Consent and Assent

Studies that involve children or cognitively impaired individuals make use of the assent process. Assent means the individual agrees to participate. A parent or legally authorized representative (LOR) grants the consent for the individual to participate.

When requesting assent, speak directly to the individual you are inviting to participate and describe the study and requirements in language appropriate for that person.

In some cases, a parent or LOR may provide consent, but the individual is not interested. You must abide by the wishes of the individual. Do not allow the parent or LOR to persuade the individual to join the study.

Note: Failure to object to participation cannot be taken as assent. The individual must agree to participate.

9.3 CONCLUSIONS

When inviting someone to join a research study, you must provide all the information needed for that person to make an informed decision about whether to participate. Your IRB-approved consent form is just one piece of the consent process. Ongoing conversations between you and the participants are necessary to achieve a fully informed consent.

Before talking with your first potential participant, review the consent document and practice the consent procedure until you are comfortable explaining the study and answering questions.

REFERENCES AND RESOURCES

BOOKS

Bankert EA, Gordon BG, Hurley EA, Shriver AP. *Institutional Review Board: Management and Function* 3rd ed. Sudbury, MA: Jones and Bartlett; 2022.

Note: Part 6, Sections 6-1 through 6-10 discuss issues of informed consent.

RESOURCES

Collaborative Institutional Training Initiative (CITI): Comprehensive Guide to Informed Consent Changes
- https://about.citiprogram.org/wp-content/uploads/2018/07/Final-Rule-Material-Comprehensive-Guide-to-Informed-Consent-Changes.pdf

National Human Genome Research Institute
Special Considerations for Genomics Research (genome.gov)
- https://www.genome.gov/about-genomics/policy-issues/Informed-Consent-for-Genomics-Research/Special-Considerations-for-Genome-Research#families

United States Department of Health and Human Services; Office for Human Research Protections (OHRP)
- https://www.hhs.gov/ohrp/education-and-outreach/revised-common-rule/revised-common-rule-q-and-a/index.html
- https://www.hhs.gov/ohrp/regulations-and-policy/guidance/informed-consent/index.html

United States Food and Drug Administration (FDA) Informed Consent Guidance Sheet
- https://www.fda.gov/regulatory-information/search-fda-guidance-documents/informed-consent

World Health Organization Research Ethics Review Committee
Research Ethics Review Committee (who.int)
- https://www.who.int/groups/research-ethics-review-committee/guidelines-on-submitting-research-proposals-for-ethics-review/templates-for-informed-consent-forms

CHAPTER 10

Medical Writing: Tips for Preparing Clear, Concise Documents for Your Audience

Lynne M. Bianchi, Ph.D. and Annmarie Kutz, M.S.

Tips for Success:

> Choose words that are familiar to readers.
> Limit sentence and paragraph length.

Warning:

> Revisions are always necessary.

Key Concept: Medical science writing is a unique style that helps readers quickly process complex information.

In several chapters of this book, we advise you to write clearly, concisely, and with your audience in mind. The advice is simple enough, but many new investigators are unsure of how to accomplish these goals. To many, preparing a manuscript or other document is already daunting. Mention concerns about grammar, active voice, and the need to limit nominalizations and it is no wonder so many residents and faculty avoid writing. Yet writing is simply telling others what you already know. You merely create sentences that convey your thoughts clearly to others.

Once you start thinking about how to choose and organize your words, your writing improves. As a clinician and scientist, you spend your days problem solving; it is one of your strengths. **Writing is just another form of problem solving.** Some people are naturally more verbal than others and enjoy writing. Others have a harder time getting words onto paper. Whatever your innate writing skills, if you have thoughts worth sharing, you can learn to compose those thoughts clearly and concisely for your audience.

This chapter provides general tips on how to improve your writing. Chapters 11–14 provide specific advice for preparing **research articles**, **case reports**, **grant applications**, and **book chapters**, respectively.

Tip: Limit **the use of the word "respectively"** as it forces readers to go back and sort through information. In the above sentence, you must pause your reading to figure out which chapter covers which topic.

DOI: 10.1201/9781003126478-10

Tip: Write so the reader never has to pause and sort out what you wrote.

Hint: If you spend a little time considering the words you use and the way you put them together, you will produce a document that is easier to read, and therefore read by more people.

Note: In preparing this chapter, the authors were left wondering how much of the advice was ignored in preparing drafts of the other chapters. Of course, during the revision stages, we will go back and look for violations of advice mentioned here. It is likely there will be mistakes, even in the final publication. We apologize and remind you that even experienced writers create sentences and paragraphs that could be improved.

10.1 DEVELOP STYLE

Writing effectively in medicine and science requires you to adopt a certain style. Some would describe this style "straightforward," "to the point," or "focused." Others would describe it as boring and lacking creativity. Some would claim that medical science writing lacks style, but that is not true. The style is direct and free of excess language. **Points are presented simply and clearly so readers can quickly digest information.**

Many of us began writing without realizing we used a particular style. We followed the advice of our mentors and tried to mirror what we read in journal articles and book chapters. Only later did we understand that our writing did in fact have a unique style. As a colleague from English Literature once commented, "You scientists just get to the point. It works though." That is a good description of medical science writing: it gets to the point, and it works.

To develop the medical science style and "get to the point," it is recommended that you:

Use Shorter Words, Sentences, and Paragraphs (But Not Always)

To improve clarity, choose words that are familiar, and structure sentences and paragraphs so they are easily comprehended by readers.

Words

Familiarity aids comprehension. Shorter words tend to be more familiar, so writers are advised to use shorter words in place of longer ones.

Some authors, especially new investigators, make the mistake of using longer medical terms when shorter ones work better. They may think the longer terms sound more scholarly, but readers often find them pretentious or confusing. For example, 'swollen' usually works better than 'intumescence'.

If, however, a longer term is familiar to your audience, you should use it. For example, 'pulmonary embolism' would be preferred over 'lung clot' for some audiences.

Sentences

In general, **shorter sentences are less confusing** than longer ones. Breaking thoughts into two or more sentences can improve reader comprehension. Shorter sentences are favored in medical writing to help readers process complex information.

However, when longer sentences contain familiar words and are structured properly, they too are easily understood. For example, as illustrated by this brief, thirty-four-word sentence, you can easily incorporate relevant adjectives, adverbs, articles, conjunctions, and prepositional phrases into a sentence without concern of losing an audience familiar with grammatical terms.

Also note that too many short sentences in a row can make your writing choppy. The flow of a passage is often improved when you include some longer sentences.

Paragraphs

A paragraph is comprised of **one or more sentences focused on a single topic**. Although there is no upper limit for length, it is difficult to stay focused on a paragraph that goes on for a page or more. **Thus, shorter paragraphs help readers grasp each idea expressed**.

Shorter paragraphs are also helpful to readers skimming through material to **locate** or **re-locate main points**.

Each paragraph contains a **topic sentence.** The topic sentence can be placed anywhere in the paragraph but is often the first or final line, as these are **locations of emphasis**. Some suggest placing the topic sentence in the **first line of the paragraph** when you believe readers will accept the information you present, but in the **last line of the paragraph** if you need to first educate or convince readers of a point. In such instances, the topic sentence may begin with "Therefore" or "Thus" to further highlight your message.

Although many of us were taught that a paragraph should have more than one sentence, it is not always necessary.

Tip: Confused readers stop reading. Use familiar words, few complex sentences, and shorter paragraphs to keep readers engaged.

Omit Excess Words

We often compose sentences with unnecessary words. We may use phrases that can be reduced to a single word (*a large number of* = *many*), pointless qualifiers (*very, rather*), repetitive phrases (*final outcome, end result*) or fillers that provide no additional information (*As a matter of fact*). **Eliminating extra words and fillers improves sentence clarity**.

> Example: *As a matter of fact, there are a number of* notes in her *past history* that are *quite* surprising. (19 words)
> Many of the notes in her history are surprising. (9 words)

In this example, ten words were eliminated in the revised sentence. The original sentence includes a filler (*As a matter of fact*), an empty clause (*there are*), excess words (*a number of*), repetitive words (*past history*), and an unnecessary qualifier (*quite*).

Fillers, such as "As a matter of fact," "As already stated," "As noted," "As above," and "As such," are overused in medical science writing. Only **use fillers** to **add emphasis**, **improve** the **transition** of a passage, or **remind** a reader of an earlier point.

Empty clauses, such as "There are" and "It is," distract the reader and delay the point of the sentence.

> Example: *There are* other excess words you can eliminate.
> You can eliminate other excess words.

Our speech and writing are also filled with **phrases better stated with their one-word equivalent**. Common examples found in medical science writing include:

Excess	Concise
The majority of	Most
A number of	Many, several
A small number of	Few
In order to	To
Due to the fact that	Because
In the course of	During
In the near future	Soon
Prior to	Before
Subsequent to	After

Qualifiers, such as *very, quite, extremely,* and *rather*, are also common. Most are unnecessary and some do not make sense. In the first example sentence, it is enough to be surprised, one does not need to be *quite* surprised. If the results of your study are statistically significant, they are significant. They are not *very* significant, or *quite* significant, or *rather* significant. They are certainly not *almost* significant. Results are either statistically significant, or they are not.

Review your writing to determine which, if any, qualifiers add emphasis. Eliminate all others.

Investigators sometimes use **repetitive words** without realizing it. They report *final outcomes* or describe a patient's *past history*. Outcomes are final; history does not refer to the future. To be accurate and concise, eliminate redundant phrases such as:

Redundant	Concise
Close proximity	Proximity
Repeated again	Repeated
Time period	Period
Already reported	Reported
End result	Result
Green in color	Green
1:00 pm in the afternoon	1:00 p.m.

USE ACTIVE VOICE, EXCEPT WHEN PASSIVE VOICE WORKS BETTER

Writing is composed in either an active or a passive voice. In English, sentences are usually structured with the subject before the verb, followed by the object that is acted upon. Such sentences are said to use active voice. **Active voice emphasizes what the subject does**. Active voice is usually preferred because it tends to be **more engaging** and **easier to comprehend**.

Examples:

- I (subject) intubated (verb) the child (object).
- The foolish residents (subject) ignored (verb) the first five chapters of the book (object).
- The patients (subject) are taking (verb) the new medication (object).
- Dr. Gopal (subject) taught (verb) the class (object).

In contrast, **passive voice** focuses on who or what receives the action. Thus, the **object** of a sentence **becomes the subject.** Sentences using passive voice require additional words such as a form of **"be"** (be, am, is, are, was, were, being, or been), a **past participle** (verb form often ending in -ed), and the word **"by"**.

In the following examples, the words required to change the active voice sentences (above) to the passive voice are italicized.

Examples:

- The child (new subject) *was intubated by* me.
- The first five chapters of the book (new subject) *were ignored by* the foolish residents.
- The new medication (new subject) *is being taken by* the patients.
- The class (new subject) *was taught by* Dr. Gopal.

Although considered less engaging, there are times when the **passive voice is preferred.** If the **subject doing the action is unknown** or **is less important than the object**, passive voice is appropriate.

Passive voice is common in the **Methods** section of a research paper because the object acted on is more important than who completed the action and, in most cases, readers do not need to know who completed a task.

Examples:

Active voice: "Nursing staff took blood samples on day 1."
                  "Malini incubated the cells at 37 degrees Celsius."

Passive voice: "Blood samples were drawn on day 1 by nursing staff."
                  "The cells were incubated at 37 degrees Celsius."

Passive voice is also used to **improve the flow of a paragraph** by breaking up the monotony of too many sequential active voice sentences.

Note: Active voice is usually preferred, but passive voice is not incorrect.

WE USE FIRST-PERSON PERSONAL PRONOUNS IN MEDICAL WRITING

Students in medicine and science are often advised to avoid first-person personal pronouns when writing about their research. It is thought that such pronouns make the writing less objective. Thus, instead of writing, "We hypothesize that practice improves writing," students are encouraged to state, "The investigators hypothesize that practice improves writing."

Be assured that you can use "I," "me," "we," and "us" in your writing and not be considered arrogant or less objective. In fact, personal pronouns have been recommended in medical writing for over a century and current journals continue to encourage their use.

However, avoid strings of sentences beginning with "I" or "We" so your passage does not read like a list of personal accomplishments. As with sentence length and voice, variety often improves readability.

LIMIT NOMINALIZATIONS TO AVOID CONFUSION

Nominalizations are **verbs that have been turned into nouns**. Scientists and physicians tend to use these often in both speech and writing. For example, we have *demonstrations* of procedures and take *measurements* of protein levels.

Sentences with nominalization require additional words and are often less clear than those without. When you identify one in a sentence you have drafted, see if the structure becomes less awkward and the meaning more obvious with the nominalization removed. Often, the revised sentence works better, as with the second sentence in the examples below.

Examples:

- The *confusion* of the patient caused him to miss his appointment.
- The confused patient missed his appointment.

- He provided no *explanation* for his teaching method.
- He did not explain his teaching method.

- They completed a *demonstration* of the new surgical technique.
- They demonstrated the new surgical technique.

Some nominalizations, such as *treatment*, are so common they are usually acceptable. Other nominalizations are useful when referring to the verb in a previous sentence.

Examples:

- "We *measured* protein levels in sixteen samples. The *measurements* were similar in each."
- "Patient data were *analyzed* from 2001 to 2010. The *analysis* revealed ..."

Hint: Words that end in *-ion*, *-ment*, *-ence*, and *-al* are often nominalizations.

USE INCLUSIVE AND PERSON-FIRST LANGUAGE

Inclusive language means writing in a way that does not exclude a particular group based on characteristics such as gender, race, ethnicity, or ability.

To be inclusive, we use **terms that represent more than one gender**. For example, we say *chairperson* in place of *chairman* to avoid the impression that only males lead a committee or department. We use *different sex* instead of *opposite sex* to acknowledge gender is a spectrum rather than binary.

Pronouns should also reflect inclusivity. He/him/his are the traditional male pronouns and she/her/hers the traditional female pronouns. Some authors indicate both genders by using combinations such as *he/she* or *s/he*. Other authors use male and female pronouns in alternating passages, while others use the singular, gender-neutral pronouns *they/their/theirs*.

Inclusive language also uses **gender-neutral nouns** (*patient, participant, student, clinician*) and avoids assumptions about family roles. For example, rather than talk of a patient's husband or wife, refer to a *spouse* or *partner*. Instead of saying a child's mother or father, use the word *parent*.

Person-first or **patient-first language** describes the person as **someone with a condition**, rather than defining the person by the condition. For example, instead of writing about "the diabetic patient," write about "*the patient with diabetes.*" Instead of "the autistic girl," say "*the girl with autism.*"

Tip: Journals usually include instructions to authors regarding the use of inclusive language, though admittedly, many are rather vague. Most state you should not use any language that might suggest one individual or group is superior to another based upon gender, race, ethnicity, culture, sexual orientation, age, disability, or health condition, and that writing should be free from bias and stereotypes.

Hint: Inclusive and person-first language should be used in clinical practice as well as in medical writing.

USE LATIN ABBREVIATIONS CORRECTLY *(e.g., i.e., AND et al.)*

Three Latin abbreviations are common in medical science writing: e.g., i.e., and et al.

The abbreviation "e.g." is from the Latin *exempli gratia*, meaning "**for example.**" You use it before a list of examples that represents a **subset of a larger list**.

> The student took traditional medical school courses (e.g., Gross Anatomy, Biochemistry, Histology).

The list includes some of the traditional medical school courses, but not all the courses taken in medical school.

The abbreviation "i.e." stands for the Latin *id est*, meaning "**that is.**" It is also used before a list of examples, but one that is **inclusive of all possible examples**.

> The student took her first semester medical school courses (i.e., Gross Anatomy, Histology, Biochemistry, Embryology, and Clinical Skills I).

This list includes all the first semester courses available to the student.

You also use "i.e.," to clarify the meaning of something already stated.

The student took first semester medical school courses, i.e., those offered at her medical school.

The abbreviation "et al." means "**and others.**" It is typically used when discussing a publication with more than two or three authors. For example, "The report by Martinez et al. (1999) was the first to describe this condition."

Et al. comes from the Latin *et alii* (masculine), *et aliae* (feminine) and *et alia* (neuter), referring to the nouns included in the list of "others." The abbreviation "et al." covers all these versions. Because "al" is the abbreviated word in this phrase, a period is used.

Note: The format of the abbreviations varies with publishers. Most include periods after each letter of the abbreviations "i.e.," and "e.g.," and some also place the abbreviations in italics. In some publications the period is dropped when et al is used in a sentence but included when the citation is in parentheses.

- The report by Martinez et al was the first to describe this condition.
- The report was the first to describe this condition (Martinez et al. 1999).

10.2 HELP READERS REMEMBER YOUR MESSAGES

We often use abbreviations, words, and phrases when discussing a project with colleagues. If our research focuses on BDNF, we rarely say "brain-derived neurotrophic factor." We say BDNF and everyone on the study team knows what we mean. When we talk about "the first group," we know the characteristics of those subjects. We become so familiar with our work that we sometimes forget others will not process our meaning as quickly.

To eliminate confusion and improve comprehension consider the following.

Include Only Essential Abbreviations

Medicine and science are filled with abbreviations and acronyms (abbreviations pronounced as a word). These are often helpful when taking notes and can improve reading speed. However, **abbreviations are only helpful if readers know what they mean**.

All abbreviations, including common ones, must be defined. The abbreviation is placed in parentheses after the words first appear in your document.

> Example: The patient's baseline blood pressure (BP) was recorded on the first day of the study. BP was checked daily over the next 3 weeks.

Although abbreviations can increase reading speed, having too many in a single document is rarely helpful. Readers may need to go back through your document to find a definition they cannot recall. Some will just skim over unfamiliar abbreviations without fully grasping the meaning of your sentences. In either case, readers become frustrated when they cannot follow what you are saying.

To limit reader frustration, limit abbreviations. **Include only those that are familiar, necessary, and used several times in the document**. If a term is used only two or three times, it is usually better to spell it out each time.

Tip: When preparing a manuscript to submit to a journal, check the publisher's instructions on how to format and cite abbreviations. Some journals require a table of abbreviations or a list of abbreviations in a footnote.

Hint: "Alphabet soup" is a phrase meaning a paper is filled with so many abbreviations that readers cannot make sense of what is being said. The phrase stems from a soup made with small noodles shaped like letters. Each spoonful creates a random group of letters. If someone says your document is alphabet soup, your writing lacks clarity.

Remember: Abbreviations only increase reading speed if readers are familiar with them.

Assign Meaningful Group Names

Label your study groups in a way that conveys meaning to your readers rather than using arbitrary numbers, letters, or terms. For example, for readers to understand the following sentence they must recall the differences among groups A, B, and C.

> The pain scores of group A were significantly lower than those of groups B and C.

However, if your group names convey information, readers quickly understand the sentence.

> The pain scores for the high-dose group were significantly lower than those of the mid-dose and low-dose groups.

or

> The pain scores of the 5-milligram (mg) group were significantly lower than those of the 2.5-mg and 1.25-mg groups.

LEARN TO IDENTIFY AND ELIMINATE IDIOMS: IT IS NOT ROCKET SCIENCE

Idioms are expressions that mean something unrelated to the individual words. Idioms confuse those unfamiliar with them. When someone says, "It is not rocket science," they are not referring to aerospace engineering. It is an expression that means something is not difficult. Other common idioms include *cutting edge, reinvent the wheel, up and running, a bundle of nerves, a clean bill of health,* and *alphabet soup.* These idioms are often used in speech more than in medical science writing.

However, another type of idiom, the phrasal verb, is common in medical science writing. **Phrasal verbs** are idioms that combine a verb with an adverb, a preposition, or both. To improve clarity for all readers, it is best to replace the phrasal verb with a single verb equivalent. For example:

Phrasal verb	Verb
Cut off	Limit
Clear up	Clarify, resolve
Build up	Accumulate
Zero in on	Focus
Look at	Assess

Note: Like all **idioms**, phrasal verbs may be **difficult for non-native English speakers to comprehend**. Your audience is a global one, so revise your texts accordingly.

10.3 REVISE AND REORGANIZE

Effective writing requires problem solving. As a physician, you spend your day solving problems, so you have the skills needed to revise text. You simply identify the problems and provide better alternatives.

As with every other skill, writing becomes easier and faster with practice. However, there is no escaping the need to polish your text. You will revise documents, sections of documents, paragraphs, and sentences many times before you are satisfied with the writing. **Box 10.1** offers tips to help you organize (and reorganize) text effectively. **Box 10.2** suggests strategies for making revisions.

Tip: Medical and science **journals offer writing tips in their submission guidelines**. Review these suggestions before you draft your paper.

Hint: The word and character limits imposed by publishers, conferences, and funding agencies can help you develop the skills associated with medical science writing. For example, journals have word limits for abstracts and grant applications usually have page limits. With experience, you will become adept at cutting out words and making substitutions to stay within those limits. Because the remaining words and sentences must be chosen carefully to retain meaning, the result is usually a clearer, more focused document.

Box 10.1   A Coordinator's Perspective: If Spelling and Grammar Are a Science, Organization Is an Art

Each protocol or manuscript you write will have organizational nuance that requires careful consideration. Organizing prose isn't bound by abundant rules and conventions; much of organization is stylistic judgment calls made by the author. In this way, organization can be thorny.

But don't despair. Below, I outline helpful tips for ensuring your drafts are well organized and ready for submission.

When to Organize

There are two points at which writers focus on organization: early, before they begin writing, and later, when they're almost done. I strongly recommend taking the opportunity to organize at both junctures. Doing so will produce the best results.

Organizing Early

The most popular form of early organization is creating and following an outline. **Outlines** guide and bring efficiency to the writing process. To create one, start by listing titles. Then, add subtitles (where appropriate) and the main supporting ideas as bullet points. Once done, you'll have a tidy framework to guide you.

In academic writing, the outline is usually straightforward—Introduction, Methods, Results, Discussion. Within these sections lies your opportunity for organizing. I recommend jotting down subtitles and main ideas within each section before you start writing.

An academic manuscript outline might look like this:

Introduction

Current Literature (Subtitle)
  – Point A (Supporting point 1)
  – Point B (Supporting point 2)
Literature Gap to Be Filled
  – Point A (Supporting point 1)
  – Point B (Supporting point 2)

Outlines are not the only option, however. Some other ideas include:

* **Color coding** text so that one color represents components of your Introduction, another color the Methods, and a third color the Discussion.
* **Numbered lists**
* **Diagrams** (Venn, for example) or flow charts
* **Columns** to visually separate ideas or information

Organizing Later

Even if you used an outline and believe your draft is well organized, it would be remiss to skip organization later in the writing process. Once your draft is written, reread it and focus on organization. Start with macro-level organization, such as the order of your subtitles and the order of your paragraphs. Do they make your writing easy to follow? Are they ordered in a logical manner? Could someone unfamiliar with your project easily understand it?

Next, examine micro-level organization. Think about sentence placement within paragraphs and sentence structure. *Should this phrase start or end this sentence? This sentence is powerful; should it be moved to the end of the paragraph for added emphasis?*

When organizing later, here are more winning strategies:

* **Give it a rest:** Do not read your draft for a few days, then go back to it with fresh eyes.
* **Role play:** Assume the role of an IRB administrator or journal reviewer. Read your work from their perspective. Try to read it with no preconceived understanding of or familiarity with the project. What questions would you have? What revisions would you request?

Writing is a fluid process that evolves as you go, even when you know the ending. Early efforts to organize provide balance and stability so you can stay on course. Later efforts sharpen and perfect your writing to improve the clarity for your audience. Both are worthwhile and necessary for a successful draft.

Box 10.2   A Coordinator's Perspective: Revision Brings Precision

The biggest writing mistake I see residents and faculty make is rushing the revision process—or skipping it altogether. Proofreading and revising are the essential, final steps of the writing process. It ensures your reader understands the content of your writing and solidifies your credibility in the reader's mind.

You may have an excellent research proposal from a clinical standpoint, but if it's plagued by verbosity, marred by typos, or your ideas are jumbled together, your reader will struggle to see the science behind the syntax. Revision ensures your writing is polished and precise.

Unsure how to revise? It's largely a two-step process:

1. **Proofread**

   Proofreading is the act of re-reading what you've written to catch mistakes and identify improvement areas. It's more about identification than fixing. When you find a mistake or perceive a weak spot in your draft, mark it.

   Many experts recommend proofreading aloud. It's an age-old trick that has endured for good reason—it works! Try it. You'll catch far more mistakes and awkward phrases when reading your draft aloud than when reading silently.

2. **Revise**

   This is the fixing stage, so roll up your sleeves. Revisit each area you marked in the proofreading stage to change it. I recommend starting with structure and organizational changes first. Once these are resolved, move on to looking at paragraphs, then sentence-level issues, then word-level changes. One strategy is to open this very chapter and find all the areas in your writing where you stray from the recommendations.

Proofreading and revising work best when performed cyclically. Proofread, revise, proofread, revise. This can continue as many times as the author feels is needed. At a certain point, however, the improvement to your writing versus the time investment of revision is no longer a sensible trade-off.

Through practice, you will execute the revision process without so much dread and, dare I say, may even come to enjoy the thrilling pursuit of a perfect draft.

10.4 CONCLUSIONS

The medical science writing style helps readers quickly process complex information. As you draft documents, think about the words you choose and how you present your information. It takes a bit of practice to convey thoughts in as few words as possible while still engaging your reader, but it is not as difficult as it may first appear. If you incorporate at least some of the tips from this chapter, your writing will be clearer and more concise. You may even discover that medical science writing is not rocket science.

REFERENCES AND RESOURCES

BOOKS

Christiansen S, Iverson C, Flanagin A, et al. *AMA Manual of Style: A Guide for Authors and Editors.* 11th ed. Oxford University Press, 2020.

Hanna M. *How to Write Better Medical Papers.* Springer, 2019.

Heineman M. *How NOT to Write a Medical Paper.* Thieme, 2016.

Lang TA. *How to Write, Publish, and Present in the Health Sciences: A Guide for Clinicians and Laboratory Researchers.* American College of Physicians, 2009.

Oberg D. *Grammar and Writing Skills for the Health Professions.* 3rd ed. Cengage Learning, 2018.

Taylor RB. *Medical Writing: A Guide for Clinicians, Educators, and Researchers.* 3rd ed. Springer, 2018.

ARTICLES

Maranhão-Filho P. Suggestions for authors of medical articles. *Arq Neuropsiquiatr.* 2017;75(2):114–116.

Lazarides MK, Gougoudi E, Papanas N. Pitfalls and misconducts in medical writing. *Int J Low Extrem Wounds.* 2019;18(4):350–353.

RESOURCES

Medical Writing March 2017, 26(1).

Includes a *Writing Better Workbook* with nine articles on how to improve writing clarity.

- https://journal.emwa.org/writing-better/

CHAPTER 11

Medical Writing: Journal Research Articles

Lynne M. Bianchi, Ph.D. and Randy Jeffrey, M.D., Ph.D.

Tips for Success:

> Incorporate advice from Chapter 10 to create a manuscript that is clear, concise, and targeted to your audience.
> Spend time designing helpful figures.
> Recognize that rejections, revisions, and resubmissions are typical stages in the publication process.

Warnings:

> Good studies, if poorly written, are returned.
> Flawed studies, if written well, are rejected.

Key Concept: Think like a reviewer as you prepare your manuscript; identify and address concerns before you submit your paper.

Publishing a paper in a medical journal is a common means of disseminating research findings. The procedures for preparing and submitting a manuscript are largely consistent across journals, making it easier to master the skills needed for success. You first select an appropriate target journal and prepare a manuscript and accompanying figures according to journal guidelines. You then submit those materials and a cover letter to the editor. If the editor agrees that the topic and study design are relevant to the journal's mission, the paper is sent to two or more peer reviewers. The editor then evaluates reviewer critiques and decides whether the paper is suitable for publication. A letter explaining the editor's decision and a copy of reviewer comments are sent to the corresponding author. If requested, the authors revise and resubmit the manuscript with a letter detailing the changes made. When the manuscript is accepted, the article is formatted for publication and several weeks or months later, the article appears in print, online, or both.

This chapter outlines typical submission requirements for research papers in medical and basic science journals. Suggestions for **selecting an appropriate journal**, **organizing text**, **designing effective figures**, **preparing a cover letter to the editor**, and **responding to reviewer comments** are provided.

DOI: 10.1201/9781003126478-11

Note: Although the basic submission procedures are the same, **each journal has specific submission and formatting requirements**. Always review the instructions for authors of your target journal to ensure text and figures are prepared correctly.

Tip: Follow all standard procedures and specific journal instructions. Manuscripts that are not prepared properly are usually sent back without review.

Hint: Understanding review criteria will help you prepare the content of your paper appropriately. Use reviewer guidelines posted on journal websites or those listed at the end of this chapter to evaluate your paper prior to submission.

11.1 PLAN BEFORE YOU WRITE

Many new investigators make the mistake of drafting a paper as soon as data are collected, without giving sufficient thought to key aspects of the process. Before you begin writing, all co-authors should meet to discuss the findings, their meaning, and how to prepare the manuscript. Discussion topics include:

Is THE STUDY READY FOR PUBLICATION?

This seems like an obvious step, but some investigators assume they should publish once all data are collected. However, there are times when even a completed study is not ready for publication, such as when data analysis reveals inconsistent findings. Always pause and reflect on what your results mean. Is there a clear message worth sharing? Do you need to collect more data first? Was there an oversight in data collection that cannot be corrected?

Never submit a manuscript if a study is incomplete or inaccurate. It wastes your time and that of the editors and reviewers. Instead, use that time to improve the study if salvageable, or move onto another project, if necessary.

Tip: If your study is not ready for publication, you can still **present your data at a local or regional conference**. Explain your intended goals, the issues you encountered, and possible next steps. You often get **helpful feedback** from others as you gain **experience presenting** and add a **scholarly activity** to your annual report and *curriculum vitae*.

Hint: Not every project is publishable, but most are presentable.

WHAT IS THE PURPOSE OF THE PAPER?

Articulating the purpose of the paper **keeps all authors focused** as the manuscript develops. Authors should agree on the **purpose** and **conclusions** of the article and outline the structure for presenting the **data** that support those conclusions. The **main message(s)** to highlight and the **figures** most helpful to illustrating the findings should be identified early in the process.

Tip: It is especially important to have clear goals and a defined structure when there are several co-authors.

Hint: Authors must work together to ensure the paper remains focused and coherent.

Remember: All authors must follow publication best practices (**Box 11.1**).

Box 11.1 Follow Publication Best Practices

Who should be an author on the manuscript? Who should be cited in the acknowledgements? Is patient consent required for a case report? Do any authors have a conflict of interest to disclose? Who are appropriate reviewers for this paper?

To address such questions and ensure standards across medical publishing, the **International Committee of Medical Journal Editors (ICMJE)** developed recommendations for authors, editors, reviewers, publishers, and journal owners (see References and Resources).

Prior to submission, preferably before the first draft of your manuscript, **review ICMJE guidelines** to ensure your paper meets standards for publication.

Remember: Follow all journal and Institutional Review Board or ethics committee instructions regarding patient consent and reporting of data (see also Chapters 8 and 9).

WHAT IS AN APPROPRIATE JOURNAL FOR THE STUDY?

Authors want to publish in journals read by those interested in their findings. Journals seek to publish articles of relevance to their readers. Thus, **the paper and the journal need to be a good fit**. This fundamental fact is often overlooked, especially by new investigators hoping to publish in the top journals of their field. What many authors fail to consider is that a great paper, if ill-suited to the journal, will not be accepted.

Identify at least a few potential journals appropriate for your study (**Box 11.2**). Keep this list in case the first one is not interested in your paper.

Tip: If you are unsure which journal on your list is best for your study, prepare a draft of the paper then choose.

Note: Submit a manuscript to one journal at a time. Most investigators know this, but some want to submit a paper to two or more journals at once to see which accepts it first. That is not allowed by journals and is a violation of publication ethics. Submit to one journal and, if it is rejected, submit to another.

Remember: It is not unusual to have to submit a paper to more than one journal. Most journals have rejection rates of over 50%, many over 70%. Space is limited in each journal issue and there are always more submissions than page space.

Box 11.2   How to Identify a Target Journal

1) **Select candidate journals**
   - List known, reputable journals in your field.
   - Use bibliographic databases such as PubMed to identify other scholarly journals.
   - Note where related studies were published; confirm the journals are reputable.
2) **Assess whether your manuscript fits the journal**
   - Review the journal mission statement to see if your study aligns with the journal's goals.
   - Check which types of articles the journal publishes (e.g., original research, clinical trials, brief communications, reviews, case reports).
   - Does your paper address a topic of interest to readers of that journal?
3) **Consider how recent publications may impact your paper**
   - Is the quality of your study on par with recently published articles?
   - Is your topic too similar to recently published papers?
   - Would your paper add new information or a different interpretation about a current topic of interest?
4) **Determine if you have the necessary funds for publication costs**
   - Are there article processing charges (APCs)?
   - Are APCs required for all published articles or only open-access articles?
   - Is there a fee for colored figures?
   - Will the publisher provide copies of the paper (reprints)?
   - How much do reprints cost?
   - Does the journal waive fees for those without funding?

Note: **Impact factor should not be the guiding principle in choosing a journal.** The impact factor estimates how often articles are cited from a given journal. It was originally developed to help librarians develop collections relevant to their users. However, over time, the impact factor became a "status symbol" for some journals. This in turn influenced how authors selected journals and some institutions began to use the numbers to evaluate job performance and tenure decisions. However, the impact factor does not mean every study published in a journal is of equal quality or is cited as often. For example, review articles are usually cited more than research articles, whereas case reports, a staple of medical literature, are cited infrequently.

Tip: Others will remember the quality of your studies more than the impact factor of a journal. Focus on publishing quality studies.

Hint: You will publish in journals with a range of impact factors during your career.

WHO IS THE TARGET AUDIENCE?

Once a target journal is selected, think about who reads that journal and target your writing to that audience. There are subtle differences in how you approach writing for a subspecialty journal *versus* a broader medical journal. For example, the terms you define, the procedures you explain, and the results you emphasize may be different for one journal *versus* another.

Tip: When resubmitting your paper to another journal, revise the text to the new target audience and format the article and figures according to that journal's guidelines.

11.2 DRAFT EACH SECTION OF THE ARTICLE

Medical science writing is direct and to the point, but it is not uninteresting. Every manuscript should **tell a story** with a clear beginning, middle, and end. The story must hold the readers' attention and help them focus on the meaning of your work. As you write your paper, lead readers through each section so they follow and appreciate the story you are building.

Most medical science research articles follow the **IMRaD** format, an acronym reflecting the main sections: **I**ntroduction, **M**ethods, **R**esults, and **D**iscussion. Some journals use variations of this format, such as putting methods at the end of the paper, but the same primary content is included for all papers.

To get started and make progress quickly, list the main sections of the paper and write down ideas to include in each section. Do not worry about generating full sentences or complete ideas for this initial rough draft; just put information and ideas down for each section as you think of them.

You likely have existing text to plug into these sections. You or other members of your research team have protocols, grant proposals, applications to the Institutional Review Board (IRB) or Institutional Animal Care and Use Committee (IACUC), or presentations. Find all those documents and **paste the relevant information under the appropriate section heading**. You will need to revise and polish the existing texts, but you have material to begin the first rough draft of your paper.

Note: It is helpful to keep this initial **rough draft** as a **separate file** so you can add to it as you think of new ideas. Create a second copy that becomes your

working draft. Copy passages from the rough draft into your working draft and revise as necessary.

Tip: Adapt your **critical reading skills** to prepare an easy-to-follow manuscript. Check that your manuscript includes the core content expected in each section (see Chapter 3).

Hint: **Many authors begin by writing the methods section**, in part because this information is already available and usually easy to describe. You can draft the methods at any time, even before data collection is complete.

THE INTRODUCTION: WHY WAS THE STUDY NEEDED? GET READERS CURIOUS ABOUT THE STUDY

The Introduction provides the **essential background** for readers to understand why a study is important. Your goal is to present a **balanced overview** of the literature relevant to your study, **highlighting what is known and unknown**.

As you describe the existing literature, emphasize gaps in knowledge that justify the need for your study. The background should be structured so the significance of your study becomes obvious. **Readers should identify the importance of your study** before you tell them.

End the Introduction with a **clear statement of your study goals or hypothesis** and the general approach used. You usually do not discuss results or conclusions at this stage. **Leave the reader curious to see what was found**.

Note: Some journals prefer you limit your **citations** to those from the past 10 years. This helps authors keep the introduction focused and up-to-date. However, the references you cite should be those most relevant to your study. If some key findings are from earlier papers, include them. You might also include review articles that summarize related studies.

Tip: The **length** of the Introduction is usually **three to six paragraphs**, taking up a half or a full page when published. Always look at other papers in your target journal to get a sense of how much to include in this section, as the norms may differ by discipline or subfield.

THE METHODS: HOW WAS THE STUDY DONE? TELL READERS THE STEPS NECESSARY TO REPLICATE THE STUDY

The Methods section, often called Materials and Methods, is the **recipe** for your study. This section explains **how the study was conducted**, including **how the data were obtained, recorded,** and **analyzed**. All the details necessary for readers to interpret the findings and to replicate the study should be included.

The specific information you include will depend, in part, on the type of study. What you describe for a clinical human subjects study will be different from that for a basic science animal study. However, for all studies you will **indicate the equipment, reagents, instruments, questionnaires, surveys,** or **other materials used**. If pertinent, describe experimental and control groups, indicate how you determined sample size, list inclusion and exclusion criteria, explain procedures for limiting bias, and state which statistical methods were used. Be sure to include any calibration, validation, or screening methods and a statement about IRB or IACUC approval, if applicable.

For common methods, you might **cite another paper that details the technique, but first confirm that the methods were the same as those you used**. If necessary, describe the modifications you made to the existing protocol. For example, "Biopsy samples were processed as in Liu et al (2002), except that tissues were fixed in 10 percent formalin rather than 4 percent paraformaldehyde."

Some journals require **subheadings** within the Methods section (e.g., subjects, equipment and materials, data analysis, and statistics) and most have a preferred format for reporting **sources of materials**, reagents, and equipment. For example, some ask for the company name, city, state, and country to be placed in parentheses after the name of the item, while others ask for details to be placed in a footnote or as online supplemental information. Check the author instructions listed for your target journal.

Some authors underestimate the importance of the Methods section. To appreciate why this content is crucial to the success of your paper, **think about papers that failed to provide sufficient information**. Perhaps you questioned a finding because it was unclear how data were collected. Maybe you wanted to use a similar approach, but information was lacking on how to do so. Perhaps a paper referenced a technique, but when you found the cited paper, the methods were incomplete.

Write your methods to include the information others may seek. Ask colleagues to review your draft to identify areas that are missing or unclear.

Remember: Most readers will not attempt to replicate your study, but they need to understand your methods to interpret your results and conclusions. **If readers cannot follow what you did, they cannot appreciate your work**.

Tip: Check how the Materials and Methods are included in your target journal. Some journals publish an abridged version in the paper, with the detailed methods available in online supplemental information.

Results: What Did the Study Reveal? Give Readers the Facts about What You Found

This section reports the study results in an **unbiased manner**. The goal is to present your findings for others to interpret. Be careful not to emphasize findings that support your study objectives while downplaying others. Include all results, even those that are inconclusive.

To aid reader comprehension, present the results in a logical order and, to the extent possible, keep the order the same as in the Methods. Statistical approaches are usually described only once at the end of the Methods section; however, you should include the outcome of statistical analyses with each result reported.

The Results section includes **figures**. Many readers will look at the figures before reading the text, so be certain to choose formats and content that effectively illustrate your data (**Box 11.3**). For example, use **tables** and **graphs** to **summarize information** and **images** to show **examples of observations**.

When describing a figure in the text, make a summary statement indicating what the figure shows, but do not state everything shown in the figure. The **text and figures should complement one another, not repeat one another**.

When referring to a figure, **emphasize the result you are illustrating rather than the figure number**. For example, *"Subjects in the control group did not gain weight (Figure 1)"* highlights the message better than *"As shown in Figure 1, subjects in the control group did not gain weight."*

Write **figure legends** that are **clear** and **specific** to what is shown. Figure legends stating "Results of the first experiment" or "Summary of data" are not informative. Readers should never have to search the text to decode a figure legend. Stating, "Participants who exercised for 60 minutes daily (solid bars) had fewer hours of disrupted sleep (2.1 hours ± SD 0.2 hours) than those who exercised for 10 minutes per day (open bars; 4.6 hours ± SD 0.3 hours; p=0.003)" provides the information needed to understand what is shown in a bar graph.

Generally, this section **does *not* include explanations of what the results mean**. Interpretations of data are offered in the Discussion section. An exception to this convention is articles with a combined results and discussion section, a format some journals require for brief reports and case studies.

Remember: **The results are telling you something relevant to the question that was asked**. It may not be what you expected, it may not make sense to you at the time, but if the study was designed and conducted properly the results have meaning. Presenting data in an unbiased manner lets others think about what the data might mean.

Note: A seemingly incongruent finding in your study may be a key piece of information needed to interpret another study.

Tip: If a figure illustrates information that is easily explained in text, it is probably not needed.

Box 11.3 Create Effective Images, Graphs, and Tables

Authors often overlook the importance of creating figures that readily convey meaning to readers. Before preparing a figure, **consider what is most important for readers to notice**. Do you want them to see the differences between groups or patterns that emerged over time? Is there essential information shown in a patient radiograph or tissue sample?

You may need to try more than one format before settling on the best option. For example, if a table is difficult to decipher quickly, a graph might work better. As you consider different formats, follow these general guidelines:

1) **To provide examples of your observations, use images**

Images are used to **display representative examples** of your observations. Common formats in medical journals include photomicrographs and de-identified patient radiographs, scans, and photographs.

Choose images that clearly and accurately illustrate your findings. It is acceptable to **select the best image**, providing it represents a **typical example**. For instance, authors usually pick a microscopy image with the best focus and staining. If the same information is found on the other slides, this is allowed because the goal is for readers to see the essential information.

Improving the quality of a representative image is also permitted, but you *cannot* **alter** the **information** presented. For example, you might crop out extraneous areas of a patient scan to draw readers attention to the areas of interest. You might alter the contrast across the entire image to make structures more visible. However, you cannot crop out areas with information you prefer not to show or to selectively alter the contrast in areas you want to emphasize.

To give readers a sense of the variability observed, it may be helpful to show examples from the best, typical, and worst-case categories.

Note: Always **apply the same modifications to all images**, including control conditions.

Tip: **Save the original image and keep notes on every modification you make.** You will need to report these as part of your methods and journals may request your original files.

Hint: When preparing patient images, *remove* identifying information from the image. If a computer program is used to block out identifiers, by placing a shaded box over the text, for example, the information can become exposed during the electronic submission or publication processes.

Warning: Altering an image to enhance or suppress information is a form of **data manipulation** and a reason for rejection of a submitted manuscript or retraction of a published paper. **As a co-author, you are responsible for the integrity of figures, even if you do not create them.** Always know how figures were produced and confirm they accurately reflect the data.

2) To provide readers with details to ponder, use tables

A well-designed table helps readers **summarize data quickly** and **draw conclusions** about the findings. Tables are best used to display **information not as easily processed as text**. For example, demographic information and test results from five patient groups would be easier to digest in a table than in a paragraph.

Tip: To help readers process the data easily, organize tables with the most relevant information at the top and put any information you want readers to compare side-by-side.

3) To help the reader process the data, use graphs

Graphs help readers **synthesize results quickly**, provided the design fits the data and the intended message. Some graphs are better suited for summarizing categorical or continuous variables; some display trends over time, others highlight differences between groups (**Table 11.1**). If you are unsure which style captures your message best, prepare two or three different graphs, then look at them from a distance. What stands out the most in each? Which graph would readers interpret most easily? Ask colleagues for their opinions and comments. You may be surprised by what others see (or fail to see) in a graph.

Once the format of your graph is selected, **spend some time optimizing the display**. Make the font size clear and easy to read. Arrange bars, boxes, lines, or dots so they are spaced appropriately. Make sure the X and Y **axes** are clearly **labeled** and **scaled** correctly. Limit any segments, or tick marks, to those necessary. To be impactful, a graph must be **uncluttered** and easy to follow.

Note: Bar and column graphs are common in the sciences. However, other graphs, such as box and whisker plots, are often preferred because they provide more information, such as confidence intervals.

Tip: Like other figures, graphs will be resized to fit the journal page. Make sure you can still see the details and read the labels if shrunk to less than half the original size.

4) To summarize complex points, use illustrations or schematics

At times, it is helpful to include drawings to **illustrate key points**. Textbooks are filled with illustrations and diagrams that help us visualize what is being discussed. Most journal articles do not have illustrations, but if you find they would be helpful, work with an experienced illustrator or colleague to develop **professional quality** illustrations that accurately represent your data.

Warning: Do not create a drawing that misleads readers. Illustrations must be based on your data or existing knowledge. If you are illustrating a proposed mechanism, make that clear to readers.

Note: There are several books, articles, and websites that provide advice on how to prepare effective tables, graphs, images, and illustrations. Journals also provide instructions on how to prepare figures that meet their publication requirements. See also References and Resources listed at the end of this chapter.

Table 11.1 Examples of Figures Commonly Used for Categorical, Discrete, and Continuous Variables

Figure Type	Categorical Data (Qualitative)	Discrete Data (Quantitative)	Continuous Data (Quantitative)	Uses	Limitations
Column or bar graph	✓	✓	✓	Compare single values. Show distribution across groups. Show trends.	Not as informative with regard to distribution within each group.
Dot plot	✓	✓	✓	Show single data points for each group or category. Show distributions across groups.	Difficult to create or read if there are several data points.
Stacked column or stacked bar graph	✓	✓		Compare characteristics in and between groups.	Difficult to see distribution in each segment of the stack. Best when only few groups represented.
Pie chart or circle graph	✓	✓		Compares parts of a whole.	Information often easier to understand with bar graph or table.
Histogram			✓	Show distribution of large data set.	Not good for comparing multiple groups.
Box and whisker plot			✓	Summarize data with confidence intervals. Show outliers.	Lose individual responses. Best for summary of large data sets.
Line graph			✓	Show trends and relationships over time.	Might give mistaken impression of data between points. Difficult to read if more than 5–7 groups.
Scatter plot			✓	Show all data points. Can help visualize relationships or correlations.	Can only compare two continuous variables.

Checkmarks indicate formats appropriate for each data type.

DISCUSSION: SO WHAT? EXPLAIN WHAT YOUR RESULTS MEAN, WHAT THEY DO NOT MEAN, AND HOW THEY RELATE TO OTHER WORK

The final section of a paper interprets the data and explains how the results fit with existing knowledge.

Begin with primary outcomes, then continue in the order presented in the Results section. Presenting data in the same order usually aids comprehension. However, if the clarity of the Discussion is improved by altering the sequence, do so.

A **study can only answer the question it was designed to address**, and authors must be careful not to overstate the significance of their data. For example, if a study tested and found that an intervention decreased pain in patients with rheumatoid arthritis, the authors could not claim the intervention slowed disease progression. They might speculate how the intervention could impact progression and suggest future studies. However, they would not imply their study evaluated progression.

All findings reported in the Results section are discussed, if only briefly. If some results are inconclusive, appear contradictory, or differ from previous reports, propose explanations supported by your data. It is important to **be open minded regarding the interpretation and meaning of your data**, as those reading your paper will be doing the same. This will help you address potential criticisms and inadequacies of your data in advance.

Always include **limitations of the study**. Every study has weaknesses and authors should acknowledge the primary limitations. **Readers have more confidence in your work when you acknowledge unresolved issues**.

Conclude your paper with a final thought you want readers to remember. This conclusion, often called the "**take-home message**," is the main point of your story. Some journals require a separate Conclusion section after the Discussion, others do not. Whatever format is used, the **final paragraph** of a paper should **succinctly summarize what you want readers to remember about your study**.

Hint: The limitations section should not be the longest part of your Discussion.

Remember: By the end of your paper, readers should have a clear sense of what the study was about, why it was done, and what the results mean. The reader should feel the study was conducted properly and that the authors were careful, ethical, and transparent.

11.3 PREPARE THE FINAL TOUCHES: TITLE, ABSTRACT, AND KEYWORDS

Write the title, abstract, and list of keywords after your manuscript is complete. These elements are saved until the end to ensure they accurately represent the content of the paper. **The words chosen influence who finds and reads a paper**, so attention to these elements is essential.

The Title

The title should be a **specific** and **succinct** description of the study that fits the journal's specifications for format and character limits. It should be **interesting** enough to catch a reader's attention, but not overly creative or humorous. It must never exaggerate or misrepresent your findings. It is helpful to indicate the population studied (e.g., children in rural Ohio, adult male mice, transgender adolescents) so readers know if the paper is relevant to their needs.

The Abstract

The abstract provides a **brief overview** of the study and its conclusions. Most journals limit abstracts to 100-300 words. It takes time to get your entire study down to so few words, but it is a crucial step. Readers form an opinion about the study based on the content of the abstract. Therefore, it is important to **devote ample time to crafting an abstract** that is **interesting, clear**, and **informative**.

Most medical journals require abstracts to follow the **IMRaD format**, whereas basic science journals usually publish narrative abstracts without subsections. Whatever the format, the content of all abstracts is similar and mirrors that of the manuscript. The **introduction** states the topic and why the study was needed. This is covered in about two to three sentences. The **methods** indicate how the study question was addressed. Essential information such as sample size, interventions, and statistical analyses are described in three to five sentences. The primary **results** are reported in about two to three sentences, while secondary outcomes might not be mentioned or stated only briefly. The **discussion**, presented in two to four sentences, highlights the conclusions readers should note.

Hint: Think about abstracts you have read. Identify the content that makes an abstract interesting and useful to you. Replicate those elements in your abstract. Also note what irritates you about a poorly constructed abstract. Avoid those irritating characteristics when drafting your abstract.

The Keywords List

Journals typically ask for a list of four to eight **keywords** associated with your study. Many authors leave this to the last minute and then provide a few words, often those already in the title or abstract. However, authors who understand how the keywords are used take time to identify additional **words pertinent to the paper**.

Keywords are used by readers and editors to quickly identify the content of a paper. Keywords help others **identify your paper during a literature search**, so it is important to choose words likely to attract readers interested in your work.

Editors also **use the keyword list to select reviewers**. Hastily chosen keywords tangential to your study may direct your paper to a reviewer less familiar with your primary topic.

If you are unsure of which keywords to include, ask colleagues for suggestions, look at the keywords listed on papers you have cited, or use PubMed to identify medical subject headings (MeSH). You can also upload your Abstract or manuscript into MeSH on Demand to generate a list of suggested keywords (see Chapter 2).

Tip: **The point of writing a paper is to have others read it**. Include words in the title, abstract, and keywords list that make your paper discoverable.

Hint: The **Title** and **Abstract may be the only portions of your paper others read**. Make them worth reading and remembering.

11.4 INCLUDE ADDITIONAL ELEMENTS
Outside of the main content, there are usually additional elements in a manuscript, such as the complete list of references cited in your paper. Other sections are optional, or only included if applicable. Each journal specifies where and how to include such elements in the submission.

ACKNOWLEDGE HELPFUL ASSISTANTS
The Acknowledgements section is optional. It is a place to thank those who helped in some way but who did not meet criteria for authorship. You might include laboratory technicians, medical students who assisted with data collection, colleagues who commented on drafts of the manuscript, or those who provided editorial assistance.

Any acknowledgements are simple and direct, not effusive, or personal. "The authors wish to thank Aaron Gee, M.S. for assistance with data collection, Jean Victor, Ph.D. for advice on statistical analysis, and Pamela An, M.D. for helpful comments on the manuscript." You do not thank friends, family, or your department chairperson for supporting your goals.

Get permission from those you wish to acknowledge before submitting your manuscript. Most will appreciate the offer, but others may feel their role was too small or have other reasons to prefer not to be acknowledged.

CREDIT FUNDING SOURCES
The source of funding section acknowledges any agencies who provided financial support to complete the project. Support from federal agencies, private foundations, industry sponsors, and institutions are listed. The name of the sponsoring agency and grant number, if applicable, are usually provided. The

amount of funding is not listed. Be sure to follow all journal and funding agency requirements for acknowledging financial support.

DECLARE CONFLICTS OF INTEREST, REAL OR PERCEIVED

Conflicts of interest (COI) forms are typically submitted by every author on the paper. Any real or perceived conflicts related to the work or other financial activities are declared. Many authors will have no conflicts and indicate so on the form.

COI are listed with the paper so readers can make judgments about potential biases in the work. Most journals and the ICMJE provide copies of such forms online.

PROVIDE FULL CITATIONS OF ALL REFERENCES

References are listed at the end of every manuscript. Most medical journals follow the AMA (American Medical Association) style, although some journals use the APA (American Psychological Association) style or another style. The journal's instructions for authors will indicate the style to use.

With the **AMA style**, references are numbered in the order they are first discussed in the text, rather than listed alphabetically. The corresponding number is placed in the appropriate location in the text, usually in superscript or brackets, depending on journal style.

Before submitting your paper, **check the location of all citation numbers in the text**. Review your **reference list** to confirm all citations are present, complete, and formatted per journal instructions.

Tip: Many bibliographic databases download references in AMA and other common styles making it easy to compile your reference list in the correct format.

Hint: By the time you are ready to submit your manuscript, you will be tired of looking at your references. However, take the time to confirm the numbers are correct in the text and reference list. Check that your reference list is complete, and that each citation contains the required information in the proper format.

11.5 GET READY TO SUBMIT: PROOFREAD, EVALUATE, AND WRITE A HELPFUL COVER LETTER

As with other forms of writing, it is best to set your final draft aside for at least a day, preferably longer. Do this after all the figures and additional elements are completed so you evaluate the same content as will the editor and reviewers.

PROOFREAD: FIND THE MISTAKES YOU MISSED

Errors are easy to overlook when you are engrossed in preparing your paper. Each co-author should set aside a dedicated time to read through the entire manuscript without interruption. Several small mistakes, such as typographical errors, misplaced references, and incorrect figure numbers, will be found. More serious errors, such as the wrong data placed in a table column or incorrect labels on an image, may also be discovered.

Because you know what should be on the page, you tend to read what is expected rather than what is shown. It is therefore helpful to **read your paper in a different font style, size,** or **color** than the one used in your drafts. Reading **sections out of order** is another effective way to spot errors.

Any **change in appearance** disrupts your previous reading pattern and **makes it easier to spot mistakes** inadvertently glossed over in your earlier drafts.

Remember: **Proofreading is time well spent.** Errors suggest carelessness, not just in the preparation of the manuscript but in completing the study.

Tip: There should be no inconsistencies in the abstract, main text, or figures. Compare the contents of each.

Warning: Papers are returned without review if authors fail to follow journal guidelines. **Review the instructions for authors again before submitting.** Put all materials in the order specified by the journal. Check your abstract format and word count. Review section headings and citations. Confirm the size, format, and placement of all figures.

EVALUATE: THINK LIKE A REVIEWER

One of the best ways to write a strong paper is to think like a reviewer. **Review criteria** focus on the study **purpose, design, methods, data analysis, interpretation,** and **ethics.** The **quality and relevance of figures, graphs, tables, and references** are also evaluated.

Critically assess each section of the paper as you would any other article. Make sure each section contains the necessary content. Try to read as if you are unfamiliar with the study to see if you omitted any information readers need. Make sure figures are accurate, visually appealing, and clearly labeled. Check that figure legends are informative.

When available, use the journal's reviewer evaluation form to score your own paper. Some journals include checklists under the online resources for reviewers. If you cannot access the one for your target journal, use another journal's or one from the Association of American Medical Colleges (AAMC; see References and Resources). Although every journal has its own reviewer checklist, most are similar.

Tip: Use a reviewer evaluation form to assess an early draft of your paper. Note all areas that need to be addressed. Review your paper again prior to submission.

Note: **If you complete a well-designed, ethical study using appropriate methods, you will meet most of the review criteria.**

WRITE A COVER LETTER THAT HELPS THE EDITOR

Every manuscript should include a cover letter to the editor unless the journal states otherwise. In the letter, **briefly** tell the editor the **content of your paper** and why it would be of **interest to readers of that journal**. Include enough information for the editor to **identify appropriate reviewers**.

You usually do not need to write more than a paragraph. The goal is to persuade the editor that your paper is interesting enough to send to reviewers.

An example from a fictitious study:

> "Enclosed is our manuscript entitled, *"Obesity rates in adolescent females living in rural counties is lower than those from suburban areas: A retrospective analysis."* We evaluated school and health records from 5,678 females between 13 and 17 years of age, living in the midwestern United States, the largest sample size from this population examined to date. We found obesity rates were 36% lower in rural areas than in suburban areas. These results are contrary to previous studies using smaller populations in single counties. Our study provides the only known assessment of daily activities associated with decreased obesity rates. We believe our novel findings will be of interest to your readers working in the areas of adolescent health, obesity prevention, and wellness initiatives."

Your letter may also include the names, affiliations, and contact information of individuals qualified to review your manuscript. Alternatively, you might **suggest reviewers** during the online submission process. Submit at least **three names**, as it is often challenging for editors to recruit enough reviewers.

Only suggest reviewers with the expertise needed to evaluate your manuscript, and never those with an actual or perceived conflict of interest. Generally, previous mentors, co-authors, or collaborators are not appropriate. If there is a reason to include someone with a potential conflict, specify your association and why you feel the individual is an appropriate reviewer. For example, "Although Dr. Klein and I worked together during our residency, he is one of the few in our field knowledgeable about the electrical recording techniques used in the current study." The editor may or may not ask Dr. Klein to participate in the review process, but you have provided the information needed for the editor to make that decision.

In some instances, you may list someone who should *not* review your paper. This is rarely necessary and is intended to identify those with a conflict of interest. You do not simply exclude people you dislike or those you deem to be overly critical.

If you have a valid reason to request someone not review your paper, explain why. For example, "We request the paper not be reviewed by Dr. Alex Dahn as she is working in a closely related area and our manuscript includes proprietary information."

Tip: If you are unsure of who could review your paper, consider conference attendees. Whenever you present a poster, note those who express interest in your work and include them on your list of candidate reviewers.

Hint: The cover letter and abstract set the tone for how the editor is going to read the rest of your submission.

11.6 PREPARE FOR THE RESUBMISSION PROCESS

Submitting a manuscript is a major accomplishment. It represents the culmination of several weeks of writing and probably several months of data collection. Once submitted, the last thing you want to think about is having to revise your paper yet again. However, **nearly all papers require some revisions**; few, if any, are accepted as initially submitted. Therefore, be prepared to revise and resubmit your paper. You should also brace yourself for rejection, as many papers are rejected by at least one journal.

Experienced investigators know **rejections, revisions, and resubmissions are part of the publication process**. However, some new investigators are distraught when reviews come back asking for more data or an editor says the paper is not suited to the journal. Some even make the mistake of giving up without publishing the study. When faced with a rejection or request for revisions, pay attention to the advice from the editor and reviewers, then **try again**.

Revise as Requested

If the editor indicates you should make revisions and resubmit the manuscript to that journal for reconsideration, be sure to address all the concerns raised by reviewers. Send a detailed letter to the editor responding to every reviewer comment. **Indicate the changes made and where those changes are in the manuscript**. For example, "Reviewer #1 asked that we explain the rationale for the cell culture experiments. On page 3 (paragraph 2) we explain the cells were used to confirm the bioactivity of our experimental protein, a test that could not be reliably conducted *in vivo*." Reviewer #2 noted we used 'is' instead of 'are' when referring to data. We corrected those errors (pages 4, 6, 9, 11 and 14)."

If a reviewer comment is inaccurate, reply respectfully. The reader may have misunderstood or made a typographical error. For example, "Reviewer #2 stated that our study did not prove office computer keyboards promote viral spread. The reviewer is correct as our study only investigated bacterial contamination. The introduction now includes a sentence to emphasize this point (page 2, paragraph 2)."

If a reviewer is wrong about something, find a tactful way to point out the reviewer's comment was inaccurate or irrelevant to your study. Remember, the same reviewers are usually asked to read the revised manuscript, so **ignoring suggestions or insulting reviewers is never helpful**.

USE REJECTIONS TO YOUR ADVANTAGE

Many manuscripts are rejected. Some papers are rejected without review because the editor does not think the study is right for the journal. Other times, the paper will be reviewed before the editor decides not to accept the paper.

Rejections always hurt, even when you are prepared for them. It is important to remember that a rejection is **not a personal attack**, and most papers require more than one submission. If your paper is turned down by one journal, revise your manuscript and send it to the next journal on your list.

If you receive reviewer comments from a journal, **incorporate all helpful suggestions into your manuscript before submitting to the next journal**. If any comments appear irrelevant to your study, try to identify why the reviewer misinterpreted your meaning. Clarify text as needed. If reviewers agree you need to collect more data, do so before submitting to another journal. If you are unable to address any reviewer concerns, consider mentioning those as limitations of your study.

Note: Always confirm that a journal is reputable. Do not get lured into submitting to a "predatory journal" (**Box 11.4**).

Tip: Though it is common to revise and resubmit a manuscript, if, after three submissions, you continue to get feedback that there are problems with your study, the paper may not be ready for publication. Speak with experienced colleagues who will give you honest feedback.

Hint: To limit the frustration of having papers rejected, **do not send your paper to a top-tier journal if your study is not on par with others published in that journal**.

Remember: As a new investigator, you want to establish a reputation as someone who does careful, reproducible, relevant work. You may have several papers in "second tier" or "third tier" journals. **The important thing is that you publish quality work in reputable journals**.

Box 11.4   "Predatory" Journals

When deciding where to publish, **be careful not to fall into the trap of publishing in a "predatory" journal**. Such journals, also called "pseudo journals" or "fake journals," are numerous and growing. They exist solely to generate money, not publish quality medical research. Of course, all publishers want to make money; however, "real" journals follow standardized peer-review procedures and rely on editors, editorial boards, and reviewers with the necessary expertise.

Predatory journals, in contrast, do not have these standards. The editors and reviewers often have no medical or science training. Some list false editorial boards comprised of well-known experts, without the experts' knowledge. In some cases, manuscripts are not even reviewed, they are just accepted.

What are signs of a predatory journal?
1) The journal's website or submission site appears unprofessional.
2) Contact information for the editor or journal is an email address unaffiliated with a university or publishing company.
3) The name of the journal is almost identical to that of a well-known journal.
4) You receive poorly written emails requesting you submit your next article to the journal. Such emails often have multiple typographical and grammatical errors, excessive praise about your "most excellent reputation," and unusual salutations such as "Dear Professor Dr. CKGASNER MD."
5) Emails inviting you to submit to the journal come from an address not associated with the journal or an academic institution.
6) Article processing charges (APCs) or other publication fees are not listed, are difficult to locate, or are considerably higher or lower than reputable journals.

Note: Reputable journals sometimes send out announcements encouraging authors to submit their papers. These are professionally prepared, usually include images of the journal, titles of recent articles, and links to the submission site.

Warning: Always confirm the reputation of a journal *before* you submit a manuscript.

How do you avoid a predatory journal?
Search for journals in a reputable bibliographic database such as PubMed (see Chapter 2) and look for journals published by well-known publishing companies or professional societies. Consult with mentors, colleagues, and a medical librarian. Check for online lists of current predatory journals.

Note: Paying a journal **a publication fee does not make the journal predatory**. Many journals require APCs to help offset publication and online maintenance costs. The difference between reputable and predatory journals is in the **integrity of the peer-review process**.

Warning: **Avoid the temptation to publish quickly by submitting to a predatory journal**. At times you may be so tired of working on a project that you may consider submitting to any journal just to get a publication and be done. **Do not submit to a predatory journal**. Publish in a journal that others read and respect.

11.7 CONCLUSIONS
Writing a paper represents the culmination of months of work. Through your paper, you share your findings, interpret their meaning, and add knowledge to the medical field.

To make the writing processes easier and less time-consuming, stay organized throughout your study and meet regularly with co-authors and collaborators. Keep notes on everything you plan to include in the paper, including figures. As you write early drafts, use reviewer criteria to evaluate each section, figure, and figure legend so you do not omit essential content.

If a paper is rejected by one journal, incorporate reviewer feedback into the manuscript, then resubmit it to another journal. If your study is interesting, novel, ethical, and relevant, it will be published.

REFERENCES AND RESOURCES

BOOKS
Hall GM (ed.) *How to Write a Paper*. 5th ed. West Sussex: BMJ Books; 2012.
Hanna M. *How to Write Better Medical Papers*. Cham: Springer; 2019.
Heineman M. *How NOT to Write a Medical Paper*. New York, NY: Thieme; 2016.

ARTICLES
Cooper ID. How to write an original research paper (and get it published). *J Med Libr Assoc*. 2015;103(2):67–68.
Meo SA. Anatomy and physiology of a scientific paper. *Saudi J Biol Sci*. 2018;25(7):1278–1283.
Saper CB. Academic publishing, part III: How to write a research paper (so that it will be accepted) in a high-quality journal. *Ann Neurol*. 2015;77(1):8–12.

ARTICLE SERIES

Bahadoran Z, Jeddi S, Mirmiran P, Ghasemi A. The principles of biomedical scientific writing: Introduction. *Int J Endocrinol Metab.* 2018;16(4):e84795.

Bahadoran Z, Mirmiran P, Zadeh-Vakili A, et al. The principles of biomedical scientific writing: Results. *Int J Endocrinol Metab.* 2019;17(2):e92113.

Ghasemi A, Bahadoran Z, Zadeh-Vakili A, et al. The principles of biomedical scientific writing: Materials and methods. *Int J Endocrinol Metab.* 2019;17(1):e88155.

Ghasemi A, Bahadoran Z, Mirmiran P, et al. The principles of biomedical scientific writing: Discussion. *Int J Endocrinol Metab.* 2019;17(3):e95415

RESOURCES

Promoting integrity in scholarly research and its publication | COPE: Committee on Publication Ethics
- https://publicationethics.org

International Committee of Medical Journal Editors
- www.icmje.org

A Guide for Reviewers | AAMC
- https:/www.aamc.org/professional-development/affinity-groups/gea/reviewer-guide

CHAPTER 12

Medical Writing: Case Studies

Lynne M. Bianchi, Ph.D. and Trevor A. Phinney, D.O.

Tips for Success:

> Read other case reports to understand how they are written.
> Review the literature carefully. Identify similar cases and note how
>   yours is unique.
> Emphasize what your case teaches other clinicians.

Warning:

> Many journals no longer accept case reports.

Key Concept: Your purpose in sharing a case must be clear and relevant to readers of the journal.

Case studies or "cases," including case reports and case series (see Chapter 4), are a common but unique form of medical publication. They describe physician observations regarding the care of a single patient or a small group of patients. Because case studies are small, observational studies, they are ranked low on the evidence-based pyramid and in the publication hierarchy. However, case studies continue to have value and are **worth publishing when there is a clear purpose in sharing your experience with other clinicians**.

To prepare a case study, you follow much of the same advice presented in Chapters 10 and 11. You use the medical science writing style to prepare a manuscript for submission to an appropriate journal. As with research reports you craft a meaningful title, write an informative abstract, choose relevant keywords, format references according to journal guidelines, submit a conflicts of interest form, and compose a helpful cover letter to the editor.

The main differences between a case study and a research article are the purpose, format, and length. This chapter explains when and how to write a useful case study targeted to your journal of interest.

Note: Typically a **case report** describes a single patient. A **case series** describes a **small group of patients**. However, the number of patients in a case series *versus* a case report is not well defined. Some consider descriptions of more than four patients a

DOI: 10.1201/9781003126478-12

case series; others define a case series as two to ten patients. Because the methods for preparing and submitting a manuscript about a single patient and a small group of patients are similar, in this chapter the term "case study" refers to both. Check the target journal's guidelines on how to label your case.

Hint: This chapter focuses on the unique aspects of preparing and submitting a case study. Chapter 11 provides details about preparing elements common to both research articles and case studies, and should be consulted as needed.

Warning: You must follow all ethical guidelines pertaining to case studies, including documentation of **patient consent for publication**. Consult your Institutional Review Board (IRB) or ethics committee and review journal instructions. Always follow CARE guidelines (see References and Resources).

12.1 KNOW WHEN TO PUBLISH A CASE STUDY

Case studies benefit the medical community in several ways. They offer insights into patient diagnoses and care, frequently alerting other clinicians to uncommon presenting symptoms, challenging diagnoses, or viable alternative treatments. Case studies provide important educational examples for students and trainees and often identify areas in need of further investigation. Many serve as the impetus for a research study. Therefore, whenever you have an interesting case that offers a new insight, you should submit it for publication. However, it is not enough to have a case that is atypical or "odd." To be of value, the case must provide new and useful information to others.

Among the common reasons to write a case study are to present:

- Characteristics of a new disease or condition
- Characteristics of an uncommon disease or condition
- A challenging differential diagnosis
- An atypical presentation or unusual etiology of a known disease or condition
- Atypical findings that suggest the need to broaden the differential diagnosis
- Unreported benefits of an existing medication or treatment
- Adverse side effects from an existing medication or treatment
- A new or improved treatment protocol, procedure, or technique
- Consequences of mistakes in diagnosis or treatment

When you encounter a case you think may be worth sharing, first **consider how the case will benefit other clinicians** or **patient care**. Articulate the take-home message you want to share.

If you struggle to identify what your case has to offer others, it may not be as interesting as you initially thought. Note, too, early in your career, many cases will seem interesting and unusual simply because they vary from the standard presentation you learned in medical school or represent rarely observed conditions. **Always review the literature and discuss the case with mentors to determine what, if anything, is unique about your case**.

Note: Understandably, most authors prefer to write reports highlighting benefits of a new treatment or procedure. However, sharing mistakes can also benefit other clinicians and protect patients. Consult senior members of your department on how to present such cases. As a resident, you would have a senior co-author on such a case study.

12.2 LEARN HOW TO WRITE A CASE STUDY

Perhaps the most distinguishing characteristic of a case study is its brevity. When you review the submission criteria for case studies, you will note that most journals limit the text to 1,000 to 2,500 words and typically restrict the number of figures to two or three. Many also limit the number of references cited. Learning how to convey the essential information within those boundaries can be a challenge for many writers.

The best way to appreciate the content and style of an effective case study is to **read other case studies**. You will learn what information is necessary to include and how to present your case in the space allowed. Start by reading cases in your field, and then read cases in other fields. The more you read, the easier it will be to adopt the proper style.

In reading other case studies, you will start to recognize style nuances used in different fields and subfields. You may observe that the language of some case studies is even more concise than other medical writing. For example, the use of articles, "the," "a," "an," is often limited. Instead of "*The* patient was transferred to *the* intensive care unit," the case description may state "*Patient was transferred to intensive care unit*." The use of articles varies with discipline however, so it is important to match your style to that of your field.

INCLUDE PERTINENT INFORMATION IN EACH SECTION

Case studies have a different format from research papers. Instead of the IMRaD format described in Chapter 11, most have only: **Case Report** and **Discussion** or **Introduction**, **Case Report**, and **Discussion**. Some journals use "Case Description" or "Case" in place of "Case Report." Although formats differ slightly, the content is the same.

Introduction

You begin with an **Introduction** to the characteristics of the disease or condition described in your report. You review findings of any previous studies and indicate how your report is unique. **Be specific about what is novel about your case**.

Case Description

The Case description combines the Methods and Results of your case. You will include **patient demographics**, **presenting symptoms**, **relevant history**, **tests**, or **treatments** given, and the **outcomes** of those.

Remember, patient **history is focused on material relevant to the case**. Details of unrelated medical history are not included. If your case is about complications during knee surgery, details of a patient's tonsillitis 10 years prior is not relevant. Different disciplines have different expectations of what constitutes patient history (**Box 12.1**). Consult cases in your specialty if you are unsure of what to include.

Present the information in **chronological order** so the reader follows what happened. When describing your diagnostic procedures, indicate any difficulties encountered and alternative diagnoses you considered.

Keep in mind that the goal of the case description is to **provide enough information for readers to make their own assessment** of the patient(s). Prepare the images, tables, and main text with this purpose in mind. There should be no surprise endings to your story. Presenting information to build suspense is neither desirable nor acceptable when writing a case study.

Include relevant information about **follow-up** care and **outcomes**. Readers want to know what happened to the patient. If the patient died, indicate when and the cause, if known. This lets readers know something about longer-term outcomes. As an example, a treatment might suggest a favorable outcome during the first month, but relapse or death by month 4. **Some journals require a minimum follow-up period of 6–12 months**. Check the instructions for authors for your target journal before submission to see if your case includes the requisite timeline.

Discussion

The Discussion section, as in research papers, **interprets your findings**, and **relates your case to existing literature**. You note limitations and future areas for research. Case studies often serve as preliminary data for larger studies, so it is always helpful to **point out areas that need further investigation**.

Some journals also include an optional section, **patient perspective**, in which patients explain in one or two paragraphs how they perceived symptoms, treatments, and outcomes. This section often adds insights that help other physicians diagnose and treat the reported condition.

Conclusion

Your Conclusion may be the final two to four sentences of your discussion or a separate section, depending on journal guidelines. Make this take-home message **the key teaching point from your case**.

> **Box 12.1 Faculty Perspective: Focus on Relevant History**
>
> The word "relevant" cannot be stressed enough when it comes to writing a case report or case series. In residency, we are taught to give a complete and detailed history of a patient when presenting a case to colleagues. However, much of that complete history is irrelevant to the diagnosis or condition being discussed.
>
> Neurologists love thorough histories. We tend to note every detail, including what a patient had for lunch that day. However, when preparing a case for publication, many of the details we love so much are not needed. For example, when I wrote a case report about autoimmune encephalitis, I did *not* include the patient's medical history of scoliosis and hyperlipidemia as it has nothing to do with the differential diagnosis or case at hand. I also limited details like "the patient then stayed in the hospital for 5 days." Only include the history that is **relevant to the points you are making**.
>
> What you need to consider when creating a "relevant" history is **what specific pieces of the patient's history were used in creating your differential diagnosis** and **what altered your work-up or treatment**. Case studies can be a great lesson in the art of honing presentation skills for your given specialty.

CREATE ADDITIONAL ELEMENTS THOUGHTFULLY

Your **Title** should provide a clear, succinct, and accurate description of the case presented. The title often includes the disease or condition, symptoms, tests, or interventions to alert readers to the primary content of your report. Include "A Case Report" or "A Case Series" after your main title unless instructed otherwise by the journal.

As noted in Chapter 11, you choose **keywords** that help an editor identify appropriate reviewers for your topic and help readers find your report during a literature search. Include any alternative names of the disease or condition you are reporting. Some conditions may be known by both formal and colloquial terms (myocardial infarction, heart attack). Others are known by descriptive terms and the names of the individual who first described it (expressive aphasia, Broca's aphasia). Choose words to help others find your case study.

As with research articles, you include any **acknowledgments** and **funding sources**. Format the **references** as per journal specifications and, if indicated by the journal, include a signed **conflict of interest form** from each author.

A unique element of a case study is documented patient consent. You must obtain written consent from the patient or the patient's legally authorized representative before submitting your report. Some journals provide a consent form to use. Template consent forms are also available online and your IRB may offer standardized forms to use. To protect patient confidentiality, the signed form is not submitted to the journal. However, you must acknowledge that you have a signed consent form and store the form in a secure location in the event you are asked for it.

Some journals continue to accept case studies without patient consent provided there is **no identifying information in the report**. Identifying information includes demographic descriptions and imaging. If you are in a small community or the case is highly unusual, it may be difficult to eliminate identifying information and, therefore, written patient consent is advised. Further, if you include any images of the patient's face, even if partially obscured, you will likely need written consent.

Remember: Like research reports, **your case study tells a story**. Write so that readers become engaged with the case, interested in the diagnosis and treatment processes, and curious to find out what happened to the patient(s).

Note: Some journals publish cases in other formats. For example, some focus on images used in diagnosis. Others publish cases to use as educational tools by including questions related to differential diagnosis, tests, treatments, and next steps.

Tip: If you dread writing research reports but enjoy teaching, consider writing cases in one of the educational formats. You will have both **teaching materials and a publication**.

Tip: Case studies should be accessible to a wide audience and easily followed by clinicians with various levels of expertise. To improve accessibility, **write as if addressing a physician in another specialty**.

Hint: Think about cases you read that were interesting and easy to follow; model yours after those.

12.3 DECIDE WHERE TO PUBLISH A CASE STUDY
When you have a case worth publishing, find a journal that accepts case studies. Be aware that **many journals no longer publish case reports**. Others publish only a few that meet stringent criteria and, even among those, many submissions are sent back without review.

There are several reasons journals no longer publish case studies. Case studies are at the bottom of the evidence-based pyramid, they take journal space that could be devoted to other article formats, and they can lower the journal's "impact factor" because they usually are not cited as often as other articles. Yet, there is still a need for high-quality case studies. To accommodate this need, some prominent **journals have "spin-off" or "sister" journals dedicated to cases**. Many of the current case study journals are only available online.

It is advantageous to **outline the information you would like to include** before deciding where to submit your paper. Check a target **journal's requirements** for content and length. Note how many figures and tables are permitted. Consider whether the restrictions work for the content you need to present.

Once you identify a target journal, **look at recent issues** to check whether a case on the same topic was published in the past year. If your case is not substantially different from a recent publication, it may be rejected by that journal simply because journals seek to publish a variety of unique cases. An exception would be if your case is about an emerging disease related to the journal's focus.

Note: As with other journal articles, there may be **article processing charges** (APCs) ranging from a few hundred to a few thousand dollars or more. Most online case report journals have APCs. Always check the APC prior to submitting and make sure the cost is within your department's budget.

Tip: Some publishers offer **discounts** to authors without external funding and most **waive fees** for authors from low-income countries.

Remember: **Do not publish in a predatory journal** (see Chapter 11, Box 11.4). Look for journals from known publishing companies or professional societies, and check whether the journal is listed in PubMed or another vetted database.

12.4 GET READY TO SUBMIT: PROOFREAD, EVALUATE, AND WRITE A HELPFUL COVER LETTER

CAREFULLY PROOFREAD

As noted in Chapter 11, you should set your manuscript aside for at least one day, then proofread when you have time to focus. Changing the font style, size, or color increases the likelihood of finding errors you glossed over in earlier drafts. Reading in a different location is also beneficial. The purpose is to break your familiarity with the document, so you read it in a different manner than when you wrote it. Anything that changes how you process the content helps you spot mistakes.

EVALUATE LIKE A REVIEWER

After correcting all errors, review your paper as the reviewers will. **Key considerations** in reviewing a case study are the **novelty** and **purpose of sharing the case**, the clarity and completeness of the **case description**, evidence of **ethical treatment** of patient(s), and the **potential impact on clinical practice**. Use available reviewer checklists to assist you in scoring your paper. Many journals post them online. If your journal does not post one, look at another journal. The basic criteria will be the same.

Note: Reviewers evaluate evidence that patients were treated appropriately, safely, and with consent.

Tip: If you report any practices that vary from standard of care, explain why you did so.

WRITE A COVER LETTER THE EDITOR WANTS TO READ

You include a **cover letter** to the editor, **briefly describing your case, why it is unique**, and **what it offers other clinicians**. Editors get many, many case studies to evaluate so you need to be clear why your case is interesting and valuable to others. You cannot overstate the findings but present the case in a way that helps the editor recognize why yours is worth sending out for review.

Remember: Novelty may refer to the condition or some aspect of patient diagnosis, treatment, or side effects. Whatever novel findings you present, there needs to be a clear reason why other clinicians would want to know about your case.

Warning: It is likely that you will submit your case study to more than one journal before it is accepted. At times, your manuscript will be sent back without review because the editor did not deem it right for the journal. Other times, the case will be reviewed, then rejected by the journal. That does not mean your case is not interesting enough to publish. As with research papers, take the reviewers' feedback into account and revise your manuscript before submitting to another journal

Note: Have a clear message that is useful to other clinicians. The relevancy of your lesson is a key factor in any review process.

Tip: Not all cases are as interesting and unique as the authors believe. If multiple reviews indicate your case is not as novel as you thought, it may be better suited as an educational lesson for your department.

Hint: Whether published or not, **present your case at a local or regional conference**. This allows you to share the lessons of the case with others, gain presentation experience, and add a scholarly activity to your annual department report and *curriculum vitae.*

12.5 CONCLUSIONS

Case reports and case series are important contributions to the medical literature. They provide new information and insights into patient care. They are often used in medical education to highlight aspects of diagnosis and treatment.

You will encounter many interesting and unusual cases in your career. Present and publish those that offer helpful information to other clinicians.

REFERENCES AND RESOURCES

ARTICLES

Florek AG, Dellavalle RP. Case reports in medical education: A platform for training medical students, residents, and fellows in scientific writing and critical thinking. *J Med Case Rep.* 2016;10:86.

Garg R, Lakhan SE, Dhanasekaran AK. How to review a case report. *J Med Case Rep.* 2016;10:88.

Juyal D, Thaledi S, Thawani V. Writing patient case reports for publication. *Educ Health (Abingdon).* 2013;26(2):126–129.

Riley DS, Barber MS, Kienle GS, et al. CARE guidelines for case reports: Explanation and elaboration document. *J Clin Epidemiol.* 2017;89:218–235.

Rison RA. A guide to writing case reports for the Journal of Medical Case Reports and BioMed Central Research Notes. *J Med Case Rep.* 2013;7:239.

RESOURCES

CARE (*Case report*) Guidelines
- www.care-statement.org

Example consent form template Taylor & Francis
- https://authorservices.taylorandfrancis.com/wp-content/uploads/2016/03/Patient-consent-form.pdf

CHAPTER 13

Writing Successful Grant Proposals to Fit the Mission of the Funding Agency

Lynne M. Bianchi, Ph.D. and Kristin A. Juhasz, D.O.

Tips for Success:

> Identify intriguing questions and appropriate methods to address them.
> Align project goals with the funding agency's mission.

Warnings:

> Grant funding is very competitive.
> Good ideas, when poorly presented, receive no funding.
> Bad ideas, when presented well, receive no funding.

Key Concept: Proposals must describe feasible and worthwhile projects targeted to the funding goals of the sponsoring agency.

Research projects often require financial resources beyond those provided by a department or program. Some projects require money for supplies or equipment. Some need funds to reimburse participants or pay research assistants. When a project requires additional financial support, investigators can apply for grant funds from institutional, private, or federal sources. Research grants range from a few hundred dollars to more than a million dollars.

All agencies, whether private or federal, award grants that support their mission. Thus, **a key to obtaining grant funding is to propose projects that fit the goals of the funding agency**. No matter how good the ideas and research plans, if the project does not align with the mission of the agency, a grant will not be awarded.

Grant proposal writing is different from other kinds of writing you will do in your career. Your writing must **convey enthusiasm** as you emphasize the **novelty** of your work and highlight its **significance** to the field, funding agency, and broader community. You must **persuade** others to share your vision.

To be successful in the competitive world of grant funding, each section of the application must demonstrate your competence and effectively address review criteria. The first section of this chapter explains how to present content and

DOI: 10.1201/9781003126478-13

illustrate how your work fits the mission of the funding agency. The second section describes the review process and the role of the review panel. Knowing how grant applications are reviewed will help you prepare successful proposals.

Note: Many people say they submit a grant. However, a grant is the money awarded when a funding agency deems a proposed project worthy of funding. You write a **proposal**, you submit an **application**, and, if done well, you receive a **grant**.

Tip: Your institution or professional society may award **grants to support resident or faculty research**. These smaller grants, called "seed money," are enough to launch a small project or collect enough data to justify a larger award from the same or a different agency.

Hint: Do not dismiss opportunities to apply for smaller grants. Success with small grants tells subsequent agencies you are worth the investment.

13.1 UNDERSTAND HOW TO PRESENT THE ELEMENTS OF AN APPLICATION

A grant application includes a **proposal** that details your research plans, **supporting documents** that describe the resources and personnel available to complete the work, and a detailed, realistic **budget** that is clearly tied to the planned work. Throughout the application, you must **demonstrate you have the skills and resources necessary** to conduct the proposed work. This message is reinforced in your preliminary data, methods, and supporting documents.

The elements and style of a grant application are a bit different from most other writing you do, so it is important to understand expectations and conventions.

Whether you are a resident or faculty member, work with an experienced **mentor** when applying for your first grants. Small differences in the way materials are prepared can have a big impact on the funding outcome. To make the most of a mentorship relationship, follow the advice in **Box 13.1**.

Tip: Read **examples of colleagues' grant applications**. If possible, compare funded and unfunded applications.

Box 13.1   Faculty Perspective: Mentorship during Residency

As a resident, I attended an Emergency Medicine Basic Research Skills (EMBRS) workshop where I learned about developing research projects and preparing grant proposals. An especially valuable part of the workshop was the opportunity to work with a mentor. The relationship I developed with my assigned mentor proved invaluable in launching my research program as a junior faculty member. I encourage other new investigators to identify and work with a supportive mentor.

Many professional organizations and residency programs offer mentorship opportunities to residents interested in building a research career. If a formal mentorship program is not available in your area, reach out to others at your institution or other institutions. With the advent of virtual communication platforms, **mentorship is not limited by geographic location**.

A **supportive mentor** helps you cultivate new skills and perspectives, introduces you to others in your field, promotes your work among peers, and often serves as a collaborator on future projects. A good mentor is interested in your career progression and supports you in ways that allow you to embark on a successful, independent research career.

A supportive mentor will:

- Encourage you to define your research goals early
- Help you define and refine your objectives and goals when initiating a new project
- Create an agreement regarding time commitment, goals, data ownership, authorship
- Challenge you to higher scientific achievement
- Introduce you to other scientists within your research community
- Give you the means to become an independent researcher

New investigators should identify mentors who:

- Have similar or related research interests
- Are committed to helping you advance your career
- Will provide constructive feedback
- Will advocate for your betterment
- Are accessible for questions, concerns
- Are willing to share sample grant applications
- Are willing to help edit and re-edit (and re-edit?) your proposals and papers
- Can guide you toward appropriate funding opportunities
- Are willing to share resources if needed (e.g., equipment, patient population, statisticians)
- Are potential collaborators

A fruitful relationship requires a **committed mentee**. The mentee does the necessary work, while the mentor provides guidance and support along the way. Even a great mentor cannot force an unwilling mentee to succeed.

A committed mentee:

- Is creative and enthusiastic
- Is proactive and hard working
- Applies advice effectively

- Respects the mentor's time
- Shows respect for the scientific community by striving to do one's best work
- Appreciates and acknowledges the benefits of the mentoring relationship

Tip: Identify mentors at your institution and through professional societies.

Hint: Seek both formal and informal mentorship.

PROPOSE EXCITING PROJECTS OF INTEREST TO THE FUNDING AGENCY

Successful applicants focus on three key factors: (1) their **writing style**, (2) how their **project aims relate to the goals of the funding agency**, and (3) **the content of each section**.

The Writing Style of a Grant Proposal

Grant proposal writing requires you to "sell" your ideas. You must convey **excitement** for your work as you highlight its significance. The goal is to write so readers share your enthusiasm and agree the proposal is **important, novel**, and **feasible**.

The **language** of a grant should be **direct and confident**. State what you *will* do; indicate what the anticipated results *will* mean. This contrasts with the language of a research paper where you often discuss what your results "may" indicate or what future studies "could" test.

In contrast to other forms of medical science writing, **adjectives and qualifiers** are common in grant proposals. Use them to highlight points and generate enthusiasm. Ideas should be *very* exciting and procedures *quite* innovative. Your preliminary data are *extremely* interesting, not merely interesting. Of course, some areas are going to be less exciting and innovative than others. You cannot claim a routine histological assay or online survey is ground breaking. However, you can emphasize how these important methods are crucial to the success of your innovative project.

Note, there is a fine line between sounding confident and sounding arrogant. **The best way to avoid sounding arrogant is to provide evidence that supports your plans.** Present examples from the literature or your previous work, explain why your resources make you ideally suited to answer the questions posed, illustrate why the work is significant to others. Throughout your proposal, choose words and examples that demonstrate you know what you are doing.

You should also judiciously use <u>underlining</u>, *italics*, and **bold text** to draw the reviewer's eye to important information. Choose formatting styles that **help a reviewer**, skimming your document, **quickly grasp main points**, and **find the information** needed to prepare an evaluation.

Include **spaces between sections** and **paragraphs** to prevent the pages from becoming dense with text. Without spaces, critical sentences are easily overlooked.

Note: What you put in a grant application is up to you. The choices you make tell reviewers a lot about your thought processes and research skills. **Select text and figures that convey competence and creativity**.

Tip: Examples are important. It is not sufficient to say your team is exceptionally well-qualified; describe their skills and experience. Do not just state your work will transform your field, explain how it will do so.

Hint: Exclamation points are not the best way to convey enthusiasm. Avoid using them!!!

How the Project Aims Relate to Funding Agency Goals

It may seem obvious that one would know something about the mission of an agency and the types of projects it funds. However, many investigators fail to consider that **a proposed project must help the agency achieve its goals.** For example, a foundation supporting pediatric cancer research receives donations to support research relevant to children with cancer. The agency therefore funds worthy proposals addressing childhood cancers but does not fund proposals focused on adult cancers.

There are many sources of funding including **federal agencies** (e.g., National Institutes of Health, NIH; National Science Foundation, NSF; Department of Defense, DOD), **private foundations** (e.g., American Heart Association, Juvenile Diabetes Research Foundation, Michael J. Fox Foundation), and **professional societies**. Each agency posts announcements describing the types of projects it funds and the deadlines for application submission.

Some agencies solicit applications targeting a specific topic. These are called **requests for proposals (RFPs)**. Some agencies support what are called **investigator-initiated** or **unsolicited** applications. These address the broader interests of the agency. Most divisions of NIH and NSF accept investigator-initiated proposals. Many federal agencies sponsor projects through both RFP and investigator-initiated mechanisms.

Some funding mechanisms require a **letter of intent (LOI)** or a **preproposal**. Applicants who meet eligibility criteria and whose projects are deemed appropriate and interesting are invited to submit the full application.

Pay attention to application requirements. If there is an **RFP**, read it very carefully and note how you would address each required element in your proposal. If you are considering an **investigator-initiated proposal**, determine how your proposal addresses the agency's stated goals.

Be honest about whether your project fits the goals of the funding agency and meets all eligibility criteria, including those related to broader impacts. It is not enough for a project to almost fit, it must truly fit.

At times, you can modify your research goals to fit a funding source. Perhaps your previous work on adult cancer can be adapted to childhood cancers. If you can advance both your research program and the agency's mission, then it is worth submitting a proposal. However, if your plans barely fit the agency's mission or you need to make convoluted arguments to force your work to match, it is better to submit elsewhere.

When you have questions about application requirements or the suitability of a topic, it is usually acceptable to **contact the designated program officer**. Most agencies encourage such conversations. Program officers at NIH and NSF, for example, are there to **educate and support investigators in the application process**. Take advantage of this service, especially as a new investigator.

Whether talking in person, on the phone, or *via* email, **have specific questions ready**. The program officer will not critique your project or indicate if you are likely to get funding but can answer many of your questions and clarify aspects of the posted funding announcements. Program officers may also give advice on how to present your work most effectively. Always check the RFP or agency website for policies on how and when to contact program officers.

During a conversation with a program officer, you may realize your project idea is not appropriate for that agency. While discouraging, it saves you the time and effort of submitting an application that would be turned down. Apply any relevant advice to future applications to that or another agency.

Note: Identify several potential funding sources. Talk to mentors, colleagues, and your institution's grants or sponsored programs office. Note grant awards cited in journal articles and conference presentations to see where others received funding. Keep **a list of application deadlines** and **eligibility criteria** for those agencies likely to fund your work.

Tip: **Pursue awards targeted at your career stage**. Many professional societies and private foundations have grant programs to support resident research. Several agencies and professional societies offer new investigator awards to help faculty launch a research career. Others have funds designated for established investigators interested in adapting their expertise to a new area.

Hint: Faculty are considered "new" for a limited period and should apply for new investigator awards during their first few years.

Remember: **It is not you; it is them**. The funding agency's objectives are the primary concern. Great ideas that do not help an agency achieve its goals cannot be funded.

The Essential Content of the Proposal

The **proposal** is the primary component of any grant application. It explains your **aims** or **objectives**, provides **background** information to support your ideas, and highlights the **significance of the project**. Detailed **methods,** potential **limitations,** and **alternative approaches** are provided for each aim. **Broader impacts** of the project, such as how the work will influence education or medical care, are usually included.

Most funding agencies require the same core content. However, a given agency may use different subheadings or require additional information. Whatever sections are required, every proposal must provide the **information necessary for reviewers to accurately judge a project's significance and potential for success**. How to effectively present essential content for each section is detailed below.

Note: Most agencies specify formatting rules such as permissible font sizes, margin widths, and page limits. Many agencies reject proposals that omit necessary subheadings, go over page limits, or use a smaller font than allowed. Given the large number of applications each agency receives, there is no reason to devote time and personnel to a proposal that does not meet requirements. As many new investigators have learned the hard way, **an application that does not follow instructions may be returned without review**.

Tip: Carelessness in preparing a proposal suggests carelessness in conducting research.

Hint: **Disregarding instructions** or **omitting required content** suggests you cannot follow directions, do not think directions apply to you, or are recycling a proposal that was rejected by another agency. None of those are impressions you want to make.

Specific Aims: This brief, **one- or two-page section** succinctly outlines what you will do, why you want to do it, how you will do it, and why it matters.

The specific aims section is extremely important to the success of any grant application. Some say this is **the most important piece of your entire proposal**. If a reviewer is confused, bored, or annoyed after reading your aims, it will be difficult to capture the reviewer's interest in subsequent sections. **Reviewers**

know that, if the specific aims page is disorganized, flawed, vague, or dull, the rest of the proposal is likely to be so as well. First impressions are critical in a grant application.

The specific aims *briefly* set up the problem to be addressed. State each specific aim (objective) of your study and the approaches you will use. If using an experimental study design, articulate the specific hypothesis you will test. Explain why it is essential to conduct this research and highlight why your research team is ideally suited for the proposed project. Convey enthusiasm as you emphasize the originality and significance of the work. **This section should leave reviewers eager to hear your detailed plans**.

The aims must be clearly articulated and precise. The word *specific* tells you how to write your aims (**Box 13.2**).

Note: The **first page must be well-crafted, engaging, and intriguing**. Plan to revise this page multiple times until it is an exciting and accurate reflection of your proposal.

Tip: By the end of the first page, the reviewer should have confidence in your team, ideas, and approach.

Hint: Complete the final version of your specific aims page after the rest of the proposal is complete. Make sure your specific aims page and project description are consistent.

Box 13.2   Put the Specifics in Your Specific Aims

The specific aims are not broad, vague ideas. You must be clear and precise. Recall from Chapter 1, the process of turning your interest into a project with one clear, specific goal (Box 1.2). In that example, the broader interest was in whether hearing aids decreased cognitive decline in older adults with hearing loss. A specific aim is *not* "We will test whether hearing aids decrease cognitive decline." A specific aim *is*: "We will test the hypothesis that digital hearing aids worn daily for 6 months improve scores on the Montreal Cognitive Assessment (MoCA) in adults over age 70." In a few sentences or a short paragraph, you explain why you are using the MoCA, what the scores mean, and why you think hearing aids would change scores. Previous studies or preliminary data would be used to support both your hypothesis and approach.

Remember, reviewers can only evaluate the information you provide. Reviewers will not know how you will "test whether hearing aids decrease cognitive decline" unless you *specify* your plans.

Project description: The project description, or narrative, is the **main part of your proposal**. It covers the background, significance, preliminary data, and approach (methods) in a manner that stimulates interest and confidence in your project.

Background: The background section explains the need for your study and its importance to advancing your field. **Discuss material that builds a compelling case for why your project is important, relevant, and timely**.

A challenge to writing the background section is providing the essential information in the limited space allotted. Cover general information briefly, then expand on material related to your proposal. For example, if your study is about bladder cancer, you do not need to devote a page to the history of cancer or three paragraphs to different types of cancers. Briefly define cancer, explain anything unique or important to note about bladder cancer, then focus on the specific literature that supports your rationale and approach.

If you devote too many pages to reviewing the literature, you have wasted valuable space. Give key facts and references; define terms that may be unfamiliar to some reviewers. Demonstrate you know the background literature, but do not belabor points or review areas tangential to your goals.

Note: Conduct a thorough literature search before you begin your proposal. Review the search strategies in Chapter 2, if needed.

Tip: Many of the papers you read will never be cited in the background section. **You must read broadly to know what is essential to include.**

Hint: How you discuss the literature tells reviewers how well you understand the topic.

Significance: The significance of a project refers to its potential to impact the field, influence current thinking, and shape future studies. Significance includes a study's **broader impacts,** the additional benefits of a project, such as those related to education, training, or medical care.

The significance is usually formally stated in a short paragraph at the end of the background. However, the significance of your study should be **clearly articulated** in the specific aims, expanded upon within or after the background section, **and highlighted** at key points **throughout your project description**.

The significance of each aim, potential outcome, and broader impact must be communicated. **Reviewers will not spend time deciphering the value of your work, you must tell them**. If you do not highlight the significance of your work, it will appear there is none.

Note: As with all other areas of your application, the project's significance must be realistic.

Tip: Illustrate the importance of your project by describing significance in multiple contexts, including benefits to scientific knowledge and broader impacts.

Hint: Always include discussion of the broader impacts of your work. See examples of funded projects if you are unsure of how to address these effectively.

Preliminary data: Preliminary data help justify the need for further work. This section highlights how **your work is leading in interesting and important directions**. It should be evident why you need funding to continue investigating your intriguing findings.

Preliminary data show reviewers you have the **skills to complete the proposed work**. Agencies cannot hand out money hoping that the investigator will figure out how to conduct the work, they need evidence that the plans are likely to succeed.

How you present the preliminary data also tells others whether you **communicate results effectively**. To make a positive impression, include relevant **images, tables**, and **graphs** that are easy to read. **Pay attention to font sizes and colors.** Include color only if necessary. Remember your document may be copied in black and white or a reviewer may have color blindness. If you must use color, make sure labels indicate where each color is in your figure.

While most preliminary data are tied to the proposed project, there are times when it is advantageous to include **data from an unrelated study**. For example, if your proposed project uses electrophysiology techniques or a statistical software package that you used at a previous institution, provide a brief description of the methods, and cite a reference **to show you have the needed skills**. If there is no publication or conference abstract to cite, explain the methods and your experience in more detail. You will not devote a lot of space to discussing unrelated work but include enough information so reviewers are confident you can complete the project.

If you do not have expertise in an area, include an **experienced collaborator committed** to the **success of the project**. Report the collaborator's relevant experience and role in the proposed study. Evidence that you have worked together, even if only briefly to test a planned approach, reassures reviewers that the collaboration is likely to be fruitful.

Note: Among the most common reviewer complaints are that tables, graphs, and images are too difficult to read. **If the data are worth showing, create figures that reviewers can process easily.** If reviewers cannot understand the work you display, they cannot evaluate it positively.

Tip: Do not waste space on unimportant figures. If a figure does not add something valuable to the proposal, leave it out and use that space for meaningful text.

Hint: Reviewers consider whether a collaborator is likely to devote the necessary time and effort to a project. Only include collaborators who are committed to working with you. Do not include a well-known investigator who does not have time to assist. This form of "name dropping" does not help an application.

Approach: The approach, or methods, **details exactly what you will do**. You state your **hypotheses** or **objectives**, detail the **methods** to be used, list expected **outcomes**, describe the types of **analyses to be done**, and discuss potential **limitations or pitfalls**. You also explain **alternative approaches** you will use if something does not work as planned, and provide the anticipated **timeframe** for completing each aim, including any alternative approaches.

By the end of this section, **reviewers must agree that your methods adequately test your aims** and the work will **lead to interesting and important findings**.

For this section to be successful:

The **proposed methods must address the objectives you state**. Check that your study design and methods will gather the data necessary to answer the proposed questions. Many investigators identify interesting questions but collect data that only partially answer the questions or use an approach inappropriate for the stated goals.

The **plans for data analysis must be appropriate** given the study design, sample size, and types of data collected. Include a statistician as a consultant or collaborator, if needed.

The **success of one aim should not depend on the outcome of another**. Specific aims should be related to one another, but not dependent upon one another. The project is too risky to fund if a particular outcome is necessary for a subsequent aim to be tested. Preliminary data may help lessen concerns about such risks. However, any suggestion that the success of the project relies on specific outcomes is a concern.

Each aim should have the potential to provide interesting information no matter what the outcome. Consider what different outcomes would suggest. If your study found the opposite of what you expected, what would that mean? Many investigators become so focused on an expected outcome or "proving" a hypothesis that they never consider the meaning of alternative outcomes.

The **resources necessary to conduct the proposed work must be available**. If additional resources are required, clarify whether they are part of your funding request or that you have another means of acquiring necessary equipment, supplies, materials, or participants.

Pitfalls and alternative approaches should be given sufficient thought and attention. Reviewers need to know you have the knowledge and skills to effectively address difficulties or unexpected outcomes. It is important for reviewers to see you have considered potential problems as it provides further evidence that you are well-suited to conducting the proposed work.

At the end of this section, reviewers must be confident you will bring the project to a successful conclusion. Reviewers understand that not everything goes as planned. There will be setbacks, unanticipated difficulties, and surprising outcomes. **Reviewers must believe you will recognize and appropriately handle whatever arises**.

Note: Some experienced grant writers suggest drafting a "manuscript" of what your study would find. While the results of your actual study will differ, and you must be open to various outcomes, the process of writing what you intend to accomplish can help you focus your proposal into a well-designed, worthwhile, and feasible project. Much of the text used in such a draft can be adapted to your grant application. Thus, the time invested is not wasted.

Warning: If you do not discuss potential pitfalls and alternative approaches, reviewers will devote much of their evaluation to the project's limitations.

Tip: Funding agencies award grants for interesting projects that are likely to be completed successfully. Leave reviewers confident that no matter what the outcomes or setbacks, you will bring the project to a fruitful conclusion.

Hint: Acknowledging limitations suggests you are an expert.

Remember: Propose methods that effectively address the stated aims. Many applications are turned down because the investigator identifies an important question, builds a rationale for what work is needed, but then proposes methods that fail to address that question. Exciting and innovative ideas using *inappropriate* methods do not receive funding.

PREPARE ADDITIONAL ELEMENTS WITH CARE
Supporting information is usually included on agency forms or in an agency-defined format. These are all **part of the review process** and **should be given the same careful thought and attention as the rest of your proposal**.

Abstract

An abstract provides a short, concise overview of the proposed project. You must effectively convey the purpose, significance, and novelty of your study in just a few hundred words. The abstract, like the specific aims page, is **critical for the success of your proposal**. The content must attract and impress a broad readership, including reviewers and agency administrators.

Some agencies require one abstract for the **scientific community** and another for a **lay audience**. Spend time preparing well-crafted versions of both. Use this as an opportunity to show the importance of your work, including broader impacts, to different audiences.

Note: If you submit two abstracts, reviewers will read both. Be sure they are consistent. The wording and emphasis will be different, but the same questions, approaches, and significance must be conveyed.

Tip: Look at the agency's website for examples of abstracts from funded projects and model yours after those.

Budget and Budget Justification

Most agencies require a detailed budget and accompanying justification explaining why the funds are needed. Devote time to drafting a **realistic budget** that accurately reflects what is needed for the proposed work.

For example, if you need a piece of **equipment**, indicate the cost, and explain why it is essential for the project. Provide a quote from the company representative if requesting an expensive or unique item. When requesting funds for **supplies**, list the total amount needed for each item. Justify this total by noting the cost of a single item and how many you need. If you will offer **participant incentives or reimbursements**, explain the cost per participant and why these incentives or reimbursements are being given. If the agency funds **travel to conferences**, provide the name of conferences you plan to attend and why such travel is relevant to the proposed project. Provide estimates of travel and accommodation costs based on recent price trends. The conferences you attend should attract those most likely to be interested in the results of your project.

Note: Some applicants request the maximum amount of funding allowed, expecting a budget cut. Others request smaller amounts, hoping the agency will approve a small request. Neither approach is helpful. **Ask for the amount you need and explain why you need it.**

Tip: Proposing a **realistic budget** tells reviewers and agencies that you know what is required to successfully complete your project. It is another way to **demonstrate your expertise**.

Hint: Requesting $233.62 instead of $235.00 does not make you appear more knowledgeable. Keep your budget simple and realistic.

Remember: Requesting more or less than is needed signals you do not understand what the project entails.

Biosketch

A biosketch is a biographical form that lists the **education, training,** and relevant **experience** of all research **personnel**. Many agencies have specific forms that must be used. Most ask for a short list of publications and presentations relevant to the proposed study and many ask for a description of how one's previous work relates to the proposed project and broader impacts.

Note: A biosketch is different from a *curriculum vitae* (CV). It is an abbreviated summary that directly relates to the proposed project.

Tip: Reviewers are looking at research team members to see if they are competent to conduct the work. Make sure everyone listed on the application provides a complete and accurate biosketch.

Hint: Check all biosketches prior to submission. Poorly prepared biosketches suggest the applicant does not pay attention to team members.

Letters of Support

The funding agency usually indicates who should (and often who should not) supply a letter of support. A letter of support may be written by your **department chair** or **dean** to confirm you have the facilities, equipment, time, and other resources needed to complete the project. **Collaborators** and **consultants** often write letters to specify their roles and time commitment to the project.

Those providing letters should have read, at a minimum, a draft or outline of your application and understand what you plan to do. The details a dean needs may be different from those a collaborator needs, but both should fully understand the project purpose and resources required to complete the project.

All letters should include the name of the principal investigator and the project title. The letter should note the role of the person supplying the letter and explain why the writer supports your efforts. Like other areas of the application, **these letters must communicate excitement for the proposed work, recognition of your expertise, and confidence in your ability to successfully complete the project.**

Warning: A short, generic, uninformed letter does not help an application.

Note: Give letter writers ample time to write letters prior to the deadline. Share ideas about topics you think are important to emphasize and explain why they matter. **Review the letters supplied to make sure they are accurate and helpful to your application.**

Tip: Not everyone understands the importance of a letter of support. Whenever necessary, ask for a revised letter that includes content that better supports your application.

Hint: You can suggest topics, ideas, and words to include.

Remember: As the principal investigator, you must make sure all proposal elements, including letters of support, reflect favorably upon you and your ideas.

Glossary and List of Abbreviations

Some agencies ask for a **glossary** or **list of abbreviations**. When **thoughtfully prepared**, these sections reflect positively on the applicant and benefit readers unfamiliar with the terms encountered.

> *Glossary*: Prepare your glossary for the **non-expert** and make sure **all descriptions are clear**. Defining a technical term with other technical terms does not help. For example, "statolith is another term for otolith" adds no clarifying information.

> *List of abbreviations*: Include *all* **abbreviations used in the application**. Every abbreviation must be spelled out the first time it is used, including those you think readers will know such as BP, ICU, WBC, or AIDS. Do not abbreviate terms that are only used a few times in the proposal. **Limit abbreviations to those you use multiple times**. For example, if blood pressure (BP) is discussed throughout your proposal, define the abbreviation when it is introduced, use "BP" thereafter, and include it in your list of abbreviations. However, if you mention "blood pressure" once in the background section and once when describing an alternative approach, spell it out each time and leave it off the list of abbreviations.

Note: Abbreviations save space and increase reading speed, but only for those familiar with the terms. Too many abbreviations make reading more challenging for all readers.

Tip: **The glossary and list of abbreviations should be available but unnecessary**; write so that reviewers comprehend your proposal without referring to either. Note, however, that reviewers will look at these sections; prepare them thoughtfully to further demonstrate your competence.

Hint: Reviewers quickly develop a negative impression if a proposal is filled with abbreviations they cannot keep straight.

13.2 UNDERSTAND THE REVIEW PROCESS

The funding agency identifies review criteria and selects reviewers capable of evaluating the proposals. Proposals submitted to your institution or a private foundation may be reviewed by administrators, physicians, scientists, and community members. Larger agencies often convene panels of reviewers with expertise in associated fields.

All reviewers focus on the logic, novelty, and importance of the ideas presented. They evaluate the soundness of the methods, adequacy of the available facilities and resources, and experience of study team members. They also consider the importance of the proposed work to the mission of the agency. Reviewers usually provide scores and written comments for each section of the application using the agency-defined criteria.

The agency then weighs reviewer evaluations to decide which applicants are awarded a grant. Proposals with the best scores are considered for funding. For some agencies, the lowest scores are the best, for others highest scores are best. The number of grants awarded is determined by the agency's budget. In many cases, the amount awarded will be less than requested. Final awards are influenced by reviewer assessments, agency priorities, and available funds.

Because every agency has a limited budget, many excellent proposals are rejected. Small differences in evaluation scores often separate the excellent applications that are funded from the excellent ones that are not. **Final scores reflect how well review criteria are addressed**. Therefore, prepare your application well in advance of the deadline so you have time to evaluate your proposal thoroughly and honestly. Use information in the funding announcement and on the agency website to create a checklist of review criteria. Make necessary revisions prior to submitting your application.

To further improve your evaluation scores, prepare your application materials with the reviewers in mind. Note their breadth of expertise and write so everyone on the panel understands your proposal. Remember, **reviewers can only rate the ideas and plans described in an application**. From a reviewer's perspective, if it is not in the application, it does not exist. **Demonstrate your competence by including all necessary information in the application**.

Note: You are advised to consider the reviewers' perspective when submitting a manuscript to a journal. Whereas much of the same advice applies when submitting a grant application, there are also unique features. Proposals are evaluated for their potential, so emphasize how your methods and resources will effectively address the interesting questions you pose.

Note: The tipping point between funded and unfunded proposals is usually in the details (or lack thereof).

Tip: Before you draft your proposal, note the review criteria and composition of the review panel. Write so all reviewers easily understand and favorably evaluate your proposal.

Hint: Review your proposal after each draft so you do not omit any required information.

CONSIDER THE WORKLOAD OF THE REVIEW PANEL

Reviewers are charged with discerning projects worthy of funding. They carefully consider and score every element of the application. The panel of reviewers usually meets to discuss applications and finalize rankings. Every panel member understands the fields represented in the proposals; however, each member has expertise in certain subfields or experimental techniques.

Review panels include members with a variety of backgrounds to provide as many perspectives as possible. Each proposal is scored by at least two reviewers. If one reviewer is unfamiliar with a topic or technique, another reviewer or someone else on the panel can offer insight. However, a reviewer's area of expertise is not always critical. Good science is good science, and **experienced reviewers can identify projects that are likely to succeed**, provided the information is presented clearly. When a proposal lacks clarity, has ideas that do not fit together, involves experiments that do not make sense, or includes poorly prepared supporting documents, scores suffer accordingly.

Reviewers do not choose which applications they review; they are assigned proposals to evaluate. You must therefore present your ideas and their importance in a way that leaves every reviewer intrigued by your project, even if they are unfamiliar with or uninterested in your topic.

Keep in mind that panel members are given several proposals to review at one time. Smaller agencies may assign two or three proposals to each reviewer, larger agencies may assign ten or more. **Reviewers are volunteering time to review grant applications**. Each reviewer is adding your application to a long list of other duties. Though committed to the scientific review process and interested in the funding agency's mission, reviewers can get discouraged easily (**Box 13.3**). Thus, it is important to **write a proposal that respects a reviewer's time**.

As noted earlier in this chapter, it is helpful to selectively underline, bold, and italicize text to separate sections and draw reader's attention to important points. Tired reviewers appreciate text that helps them focus and relocate key points. The key is to **use formatting strategically and sparingly**.

Remember, writing reflects your thinking. If you cannot write about your ideas clearly, reviewers will assume you do not think clearly and quickly lose confidence in your proposal. Perhaps the most important thing to remember when preparing your proposal is that **a reviewer should never have to think**. If a reviewer must pause and sort out what you are trying to convey, you have likely lost a favorable critique. Reviewers have little patience with proposals they must decipher.

Reviewers also lose patience with applicants attempting to skirt page limits and formatting guidelines. Do not be tempted to save space by using small font sizes in graphs, cramming too much data into a figure, or adding background information into figure legends. Reviewers will not hunt for information hidden in the document. When reviewers cannot easily view figures or find information, they focus attention on applications that are easier to follow.

Many investigators claim that they do not get funding because they never know what the reviewers want. The answer is quite simple: **reviewers want** to read proposals that clearly describe **interesting questions addressed by competent investigators using appropriate methods**.

Investigators should note that **reviewers do not want** proposals with **partially developed ideas** or proposals describing projects that would add **minimal new knowledge** to the field. They especially do not want to read a poorly developed proposal submitted by an investigator hoping to get feedback to use in a resubmission.

Remember: The **easier your proposal is to follow** the **more impressed reviewers will be**.

Note: The importance of preparing well-written materials targeted to a broad audience cannot be overstated.

Tip: Not every reviewer reads the application in the order you present. **Check that every part of your application reflects favorably upon you and your ideas**.

Hint: Some reviewers wait until the last minute to read proposals. Write so those who are rushing through your application can easily understand your project.

Box 13.3   A Reviewer's Perspective: The Benefits and Frustrations of Reading Proposals

As any reviewer will tell you, it is both an honor and a burden to sit on a review panel. Like other investigators, I take the peer-review process seriously and want to contribute to my field. I enjoy reading about others ideas and hearing about emerging areas of research. Thus, serving on a review panel is something I am willing to do. However, it is on top of every other responsibility I have, and I must carve out time in my days to review each proposal. I usually review early in the morning, before my regular day begins, and on weekends.

Like other reviewers, I recognize and appreciate the effort that goes into preparing a grant proposal. I know every investigator spends time developing ideas, writing the proposal, and submitting all the required forms. The submission process alone is time consuming and often frustrating. And like reviewing, proposal writing is added to the investigator's other duties. Unless one is on sabbatical, one usually does not get released from other responsibilities to write a proposal. Thus, I begin the review process empathetic to the investigator.

However, my empathy quickly evaporates when a proposal is disorganized, and I must make notes to sort out what the investigators plan to do or figure out what the various outcomes might indicate. My opinion of the application grows less favorable the more I must do this.

Other reviewers express the same concerns about a poorly prepared proposal, and it is no coincidence that proposals lacking clarity are unsuccessful. Reviewers cannot help but assume that an investigator who submits a confusing proposal is not ready to take on the responsibility of a grant.

Successful proposals present ideas simply and clearly. **The best proposals lead a reader through each step, explaining the purpose of each experiment and what every expected and alternative outcome would mean**.

Serving on a review panel gave me a greater appreciation for the peer-review process and taught me how to better prepare proposals of my own. The experience showed me what information reviewers need to evaluate a project and how to write so others can easily grasp my plans.

Hint: Take advantage of invitations to sit on a review panel.

PERSIST TO SUCCEED

There are toys designed to pop back up whenever you push them over. No matter how many times or how hard you push, they never stay down. To be successful in obtaining grant funding, you need to be like one of those toys. Pop back up and try again whenever an application is declined. If the ideas are good, your **persistence will pay off**.

Be prepared for rejections and resubmissions. It is simply part of the process. When reviewers knock down your ideas or methods, take their criticisms into account, revise your application accordingly, and resubmit. If your ideas are not well suited to one agency, rework your proposal, and send it to one that is a better fit.

Everyone has grant proposals rejected. Some have many rejected before they get one funded, some have one funded as a new investigator then spend a few years trying to get a second award. It can be a very disheartening process, and many give up before they should. Keep in mind that **grant funding is finite, and many good proposals must be turned down**.

Use Reviews to Shape Resubmissions

When a proposal is not funded it is natural to be upset, disappointed, annoyed, or even angry with the reviewers. Spend a day or two venting about how horrible the reviews were and how the panel was comprised of people incapable of recognizing your brilliance. Once you get that out of your system, refocus, read the reviews again, and identify the points that will help you create a fundable proposal.

The **reviewer critiques provide helpful guidance**, and you should take advantage of that guidance when revising a proposal. If you decide to resubmit to a different agency, adapt the advice accordingly before submitting elsewhere.

Share the reviews with your mentor or other experienced colleagues. They can view the comments objectively, suggest how to address concerns, and offer advice on how to reply to any comments that are off topic. **Do not be embarrassed that your grant was not funded**. Every experienced investigator has grants rejected.

Note: **Always take reviewer comments into account when preparing a revised application**. Pay attention to all comments and reflect on how to use critiques to improve your proposal.

Tip: When you submit a revised application to the same funding agency, the **same reviewers are likely to critique your resubmission**. Thoughtfully and politely respond to all reviewer comments, whether you agree with them or not.

Hint: **Members of the review panel will have access to previous reviews**. Do not disregard reviewer comments, thinking that no one will notice.

Build a Reputation for Success

Bringing a smaller grant to conclusion demonstrates you conceive worthwhile ideas, design appropriate methods, and follow through on plans. Reviewers and funding agencies support those most likely to complete worthwhile projects. Therefore, the track record you build over time **demonstrates your research is worth the investment**. Success breeds success.

13.3 CONCLUSIONS

A successful grant proposal requires innovative, feasible ideas that match the goals of the funding agency. To prepare a successful application:

1) Submit a proposal that helps the funding agency achieve its goals.
2) Write so a reviewer never has to stop and think.
3) Clearly state the specific aims and their significance.
4) Identify potential difficulties and explain how you will address any issues that arise.

5) Review the application instructions after each draft to ensure all required elements are addressed.
6) Check that all supporting documents capture the importance of your proposed work.
7) Read your penultimate draft as if you were a reviewer. Revise accordingly.

REFERENCES AND RESOURCES

BOOKS
Gitlin LN, Kolanowski A, Lyons KJ. *Successful Grant Writing: Strategies for Health and Human Service Professionals*. 5th ed. New York, NY: Springer; 2020.

ARTICLES
Clark RC, Carter KF. Successful grant applications: Follow the 4 F's. *Nursing*. 2019;49(2):55–58.
Crow JM. What to do when your grant is rejected. *Nature*. 2020;578(7795):477–479.
Files DC, Hume PS, Krall J, et al. Grant writing for clinicians in training: An important career development exercise. *Chest*. 2020;157(4):932–935.
Kwok R. You can get that paper, thesis or grant written—with a little help. *Nature*. 2020;580(7801):151–153.
Monte AA, Libby AM. Introduction to the specific aims page of a grant proposal. *Acad Emerg Med*. 2018;25(9):1042–1047.
Porter R. Why academics have a hard time writing good grant proposals. *J Res Admin*. 2007; 38(2):37–43.
Seeman E. The ABC of writing a grant proposal. *Osteoporos Int*. 2015;26(6):1665–1666.
Wegener S, Katan M. Getting the first grant. *Stroke*. 2018;49(1):e7–e9.

ARTICLE SERIES
Sauer RM, Gabbi C. Grantsmanship: What? Who? How? *Eur J Intern Med*. 2018;57:22–24.
Gabbi C, Sauer RM. Grantsmanship writing tips: Background, hypothesis and aims. *Eur J Intern Med*. 2019;61:25–28.
Gabbi C, Sauer RM. Grantsmanship writing tips: The experimental design. *Eur J Intern Med*. 2019;64:21–23.
Sauer RM, Gabbi C. Grantsmanship writing tips: Significance, innovation and impact. *Eur J Intern Med*. 2019;65:26–28.

RESOURCES
POTENTIAL FUNDING SOURCES

Professional societies associated with your specialty may award for grants targeted to residents, new faculty, established investigators (e.g., Centralized Otolaryngology Research Efforts, Society for Academic Emergency Medicine, Orthopaedic Research and Education Foundation).

Private foundations supporting research related to diseases/conditions in your specialty area (e.g., juvenile diabetes, deafness, spinal cord injury).

United States Government (international applicants are eligible for many programs, see websites for details):

General Information
This site includes information on grantsmanship, eligibility, and specific funding opportunities from different agencies, including *Department of Defense, Department of Agriculture, Department of Health and Human Services, Veterans Affairs, National Science Foundation, Small Business Administration.*
- https://www.grants.gov

National Institutes of Health (part of United States Department of Health and Human Services)
This site provides information on grantsmanship, the mission and funding opportunities under each division of NIH, awards targeted to career stage, other special topics.
- https://grants.nih.gov/grants/funding/funding_program.htm

Agency for Healthcare Research and Quality (part of United States Department of Health and Human Services)
The site explains funding opportunities to support projects focused on healthcare services and delivery, and research targeting improved safety, quality, accessibility, equity, and affordability.
- https://www.ahrq.gov/funding/index.htm

CHAPTER 14

Writing Book Chapters

Lynne M. Bianchi, Ph.D. and John D. Lubahn, M.D.

Tips for Success:

> Review requirements prior to agreeing to contribute.
> Ensure you have the expertise needed and can meet all deadlines.

Warning:

> There are times when it is best to decline an invitation to write a book chapter.

Key Concept: Writing a book chapter is a unique way to contribute expertise and influence your field.

Writing a book chapter requires many of the same skills as other forms of medical science writing, yet there are also unique aspects. You are typically invited to contribute a chapter based on your expertise. Although content, structure, length, writing style, and due date are largely dictated by the book's editors, you are usually encouraged to share experiences, express opinions, and make predictions. Thus, a book chapter allows you to impact your field in novel and important ways.

Because you are invited based on your knowledge and standing in the field, it is usually considered an honor to contribute a chapter to a book. However, writing a book chapter, like every other scholarly activity, takes time. There may be periods in your career when adding a book chapter to your to-do list does not make sense.

Advice to help you decide when to accept and when to decline a book chapter invitation is provided in the first part of this chapter. The second section outlines steps to follow to produce a chapter well suited to those books you agree to contribute.

14.1 UNDERSTAND PUBLISHING PRACTICES AND EXPECTATIONS

Many books in the medical and basic sciences are published every year. Content ranges from general information for a lay audience, to introductory textbooks, to detailed specialty-focused handbooks for advanced students and practitioners.

DOI: 10.1201/9781003126478-14

Some books are written by one or a few authors with no outside contributors. Others, such as this book, are largely written by the **primary author(s)** but include **invited contributors** who author, or co-author, selected chapters. Contributors are typically given instructions regarding structure and content to ensure the invited chapters align with the rest of the book. In general, there are more guidelines when contributing to a book of this format.

Another common format, called an **edited volume**, contains chapters written by different authors around a single theme, such as development of the auditory system, emerging techniques in hand surgery, or research methods for graduate nursing students. The editors may write a chapter or two themselves but rely primarily on **content from the invited experts**. Books based on conference proceedings are also published as edited volumes, with chapters contributed by conference speakers. Editors may play a significant role in helping authors revise chapters, or may be less involved, expecting authors to revise and edit their own work.

Note: It is important to know the intended purpose, planned content, and basic organization of a proposed book before you decide whether to contribute a chapter. The role and responsibilities of the primary authors or editors should be defined.

THE INVITATION TO CONTRIBUTE

Clinicians and researchers are invited to write a book chapter based on their previous work, areas of expertise, and standing in the field. Most invitations are issued for edited volumes for which the editors seek "words of wisdom" from those knowledgeable about the topics they want covered. **If the editors recognize you as someone likely to add valuable content, you are invited to contribute a chapter**.

Colleagues, former mentors, individuals you meet at conferences, and others familiar with your work may invite you to contribute a chapter. Your career stage often influences how you are identified as a potential author (**Box 14.1**).

You typically receive an email or phone call inviting you to participate in the book project. The general purpose of the book and your contribution are outlined. If you express interest, or at least do not decline immediately, more details will follow.

Box 14.1   Invitations Based on Career Stage

As a **resident or fellow**, a senior colleague or mentor may ask you to assist with a chapter they have committed to writing. This is an educational opportunity for you to learn more about the topic and develop your writing skills. It also provides a co-authored publication with an established investigator.

At other times **early in your career**, invitations for co-authorship may come from former or current colleagues. Some may need help with a section of a chapter and ask you to contribute your expertise. Others know you are coming up for tenure and offer co-authorship to help you round out your *curriculum vitae*. Publishing with established co-authors at early-career stages can help promote your standing in the field.

As an **established clinician or investigator**, editors will contact you directly. Depending on the topic and timing of the request, you might accept the invitation, ask to include a co-author, suggest someone else, or simply decline.

Note: Your name may be suggested by someone who declined an invitation. When editors are turned down by one potential author, they may ask for names of others with similar expertise. It may seem insulting to be the second or third person invited to contribute a chapter, but, if the project is of interest and the timing works for you, it is worth accepting. One of us was "second choice" to contribute a chapter to a book that became a seminal work in the field. There is nothing insulting about that.

THE BOOK PURPOSE AND AUTHOR RESPONSIBILITIES

Before you commit to writing a chapter, **gather as much information as you can about the book**. You want to be certain you have the expertise needed to write the chapter and that the goals of the book are consistent with your interests. At minimum, you want to know the **intended purpose, target audience, topics of the other chapters, and names of other contributors**.

First, consider whether the objective of the book fits with your expertise and whether you are comfortable writing in the style necessary for the intended audience.

If the book sounds like a good fit for you, look carefully at the requirements. What is the expected **length of the chapter**? You may be given page limits, word limits, or character limits for your document. You can anticipate most chapter requests will be for about fifteen to thirty double spaced pages, excluding figures, or about 4,000–10,000 words of text. In general, chapters for textbooks are longer than those for a research proceedings book. Although the length of any chapter will vary based on the book, topic, and other criteria, these estimates let you know if the project is substantially different from a typical chapter.

Before you agree to write the chapter, try to estimate how much text it will take to cover the topic satisfactorily. If you think the defined limits are too low or too high, discuss your concerns.

Ask whether you should include **figures** and if there are **limits on the number, format, or colors**. Clarify who is responsible for creating the figures. Should you use unpublished figures from your own work or from previous publications? Can you include copyrighted figures or illustrations from others? Who is responsible for obtaining permission to use copyrighted materials? Will you need to do that on your own or will the editor or publisher help? Acquiring permission to use figures from other published sources is not that difficult, but it takes some lead time, so you want to confirm the procedures to follow.

If illustrations are requested, who will complete those? Will you create your own illustrations in a specified computer program, or will the editor have you work with an illustrator? If working with an illustrator, what types of drawings are you expected to provide? When are those due? (**Box 14.2**).

It is also helpful to **understand the role of the editors**. The editors usually identify chapter topics, set content and formatting standards, and assign deadlines. Most editors read the chapters and request revisions to create a coherent book. Some editors are very involved and give detailed feedback, whereas others are more hands-off, leaving authors to include what they feel is best. Find out what the editors of the proposed book expect of you and how much assistance, if any, they will provide. Consider whether their expectations and management style seem reasonable.

Find out if the book is under contract. Most editors will have a contract signed with a publisher and an anticipated publication date before they invite chapters from others. Sometimes, a colleague may ask for your tentative commitment to a book they are proposing to a publisher. In either case, wait until the book is under contract before you start writing. You do not want to invest time writing a chapter for a book that is never published.

In some cases, you may be asked to submit an outline of your chapter. Editors may share this with the publisher or other authors. When available, **get outlines of the other chapters** so you do not create overlapping content.

If asked to provide an outline prior to the publishing contract being finalized, consider how well you know the editors and how confident you are that the project will proceed. You do not want to devote hours preparing a chapter outline only to find out the book is never published, or that your ideas are used by someone else.

Note: If you do not know the editors, personally or by reputation, find out more about them before you agree to write. In most cases, the books will be real and the editors sincere in their efforts. When that is the case, they will be happy to share information. If they are not forthcoming with information, you should remain skeptical until you are certain the project will be completed.

Tip: There is little or no financial incentive for writing a chapter. You often get a copy of the book or reprints of your chapter. Book authors and editors receive royalties from the publisher, but they are not large. They may receive 7–15%

of the purchase price from new book sales. As many authors and editors soon discover, even when a book sells well, royalty payments work out to less than fifty cents per hour of work. **You contribute to books because you want to share knowledge about a topic of interest, not for financial gain**.

Hint: **Do not pay to have a chapter added to a book**. While there is no financial incentive to contribute, there is also no cost. Be suspicious of solicitations from editors or publishers offering to include your chapter in an upcoming book for a fee. If your content is important to the book, no one will ask you to pay to have it included.

Box 14.2 Author's Perspective: Working with an Illustrator

When debating whether to write a textbook requiring several illustrations, I was reassured by an editor that a professional illustrator would produce the figures. I only had to provide sketches and the illustrator would do the rest. That seemed easy enough until my labeled line drawings were sent back with the comment "draw exactly what you want and include all colors and labels precisely where you want them." There was clearly a miscommunication about what "provide sketches" meant. To prevent similar misunderstandings, discuss such details early in the project and put agreed practices in writing.

Note: The illustrator successfully turned my colored sketches into quality illustrations.

THE DEADLINES TO MEET

As a contributing author, you must **understand and adhere to the deadlines issued**. There are many steps involved in publishing a book. Authors write the chapters, editors review the chapters, and the publisher produces the book, often in both print and electronic formats. Everyone needs to complete assigned elements in a timely fashion for the book to be published on schedule.

The anticipated publication date is usually a year or more after you first agree to contribute. However, the actual publication date depends on how well deadlines are met. When authors turn in materials late, a book can be held up for months or even years.

You will be given a deadline to submit the chapter, and subsequent deadlines for revisions. **Consider whether you can meet the deadlines issued by the editors before agreeing to write a chapter**.

Editors and publishers expect some delays. They set target deadlines to accommodate unanticipated setbacks. However, they are planning for unanticipated setbacks, not delays of several months caused by an author who is unable or unwilling to finish a chapter on time (**Box 14.3**).

Tip: If you find you cannot meet a deadline, inform the editors as soon as you know and give a revised date for submission. If your delay is extensive, they may need to make other arrangements.

Hint: If colleagues tell you that deadlines are fluid and it does not matter when you turn in a chapter, do not believe them.

Box 14.3   Contributor's Perspective: Why Meeting Deadlines Matters

As a junior faculty member, a senior colleague once advised me not to worry about a looming chapter deadline. He explained, "I was several months late with my chapter for Dr. R's book, and it did not matter. She was just happy to have someone write the chapter." At a conference a year or so later, I met Dr. R., who recognized that I was in the same department as the tardy author. Her first statement was, "I hope you are not like your colleague. He held up our book for months! None of us will work with him again. He does not get things done on time."

Hint: Adhere to deadlines; if you are unreliable, others soon find out.

14.2 KNOW WHEN TO CONTRIBUTE A BOOK CHAPTER

Consider your interest in the project and your available time. You will always be busy. You will always have other commitments. Sometimes, it will be easy to know if it is the right time to agree to write a chapter. Other times, you may be less certain. Here are some points to consider when deciding if you should commit to the project.

HOW WOULD A CHAPTER IMPACT ONGOING PROJECTS AND LOOMING DEADLINES?

When you have a research paper or grant application to finish, it is often best to decline the invitation. **Papers and grants take priority**. Declining for such reasons is understandable and acceptable. For example, authors of this book invited a junior colleague to co-author a chapter. We valued her input and wanted to support her career by offering a scholarly activity. However, she had a grant application deadline to meet in the same timeframe. As much as we wanted her contribution, we knew her time would be better spent on the grant proposal.

When weighing whether to commit to a chapter, keep in mind the time from submission to publication. If you are trying to build your publication list, it is usually better to work on an original research article or review paper first. If, however, you are in the midst of data collection and have time to write, it may be a good time to work on a book chapter. **Having multiple publication formats in progress can ensure you produce scholarly work on a regular basis.**

Note: In general, writing a book chapter in medicine or science is not ranked as important as writing an original research article because chapters are not peer-reviewed in the same manner. If research articles are needed for tenure or promotion, you should focus your efforts accordingly.

Tip: You should never agree to a project you cannot finish in the allotted time. If you are interested in contributing but need more time, discuss a revised timeline with the editors.

You Might Accept If the Book Is Interesting and Written by Leaders in Your Field

If the book is about a topic of interest to you and includes editors or chapter authors internationally known in your field, or the book is a new edition of a well-respected volume in your field, it is usually **worth considering** having your name associated with that book.

Think about how working on the chapter would influence your ability to complete current research projects or other scholarly work. **If you can write the chapter without falling behind on other priorities, you should consider writing it.**

Tip: If helpful, enlist a reliable colleague to co-author the chapter with you. As with all publications, the contributions of each author and the order of authorship should be agreed on before the work begins.

Hint: Not every co-author is helpful. Choose your co-authors carefully.

Decline If the Book Is Not of Interest to You

Some requests to contribute a chapter will be unappealing. The book content or chapter topic may not be a primary interest of yours. The format requested may require more time than you are willing or able to commit to, or perhaps you do not enjoy writing in the style needed for the target audience.

There are many times an invitation to contribute a chapter will not be of interest to you. It is **usually better to decline** and **save your time for another project**. Weigh the pros and cons of contributing and make your decision based on what is best for you.

Note: If you decline an invitation, do so in a professional and courteous manner. Although you may not be interested in that book or topic, you will probably be interested in others. Your reputation will be influenced by how you decline offers.

Tip: Do not agree to write a chapter on a topic outside your area of expertise unless you are working with an expert co-author. The time spent learning about the topic is likely better spent on other scholarly activities.

14.3 HOW TO PREPARE A CHAPTER

Before beginning a chapter you have agreed to write, have a clear understanding of the **purpose** and goals of the book, the **target audience**, and the **preferred writing style**. Confirm what content you should include, and when materials are due.

OUTLINE THE GENERAL CONTENT BASED ON YOUR KNOWLEDGE OF THE TOPIC

First, think about what you would like to include in the chapter and identify the information you need to gather. **List the general content, main points, and figures you could include**. Think about how you might organize the information.

Your initial outline may include:

- Points and opinions you want to emphasize
- Topics that will require more detailed explanations
- Areas that may be controversial or inconclusive
- Ideas for figures and the formats of each
- Papers and authors to cite
- Areas to include in a literature search

Remember: An outline does not have to be a formal outline with Roman numerals and multiple subheadings. Draft your ideas in a format that works for you and any co-authors.

CONDUCT A THOROUGH LITERATURE SEARCH

Readers of a book chapter are relying on the authors to educate them. They expect, and need, a full account of the topic. When writing a book chapter, you must decide what is most helpful for a reader to know. Thus, you first identify and read as many relevant papers as you can find, then pick what content to include in the chapter.

Your literature search should begin by focusing on the content in your first outline and then expand based on the articles you read. As you revise your outline and draft your chapter, some of the materials you read will be cited and others will not. As with other forms of writing, **you always read more than you will ultimately discuss**.

Be sure to **include citations others would benefit from reading**. A chapter should highlight recent advances, but also include seminal papers in your field.

Note: A book chapter is not a systematic review of the literature, and you are not critiquing every paper on the topic. You must choose what content is important to your readers. Do not dismiss information that disagrees with your opinions but omit topics that stray from your main points.

Tip: Some editors indicate how many references to include at the end of your chapter. If you are not given any guidelines, expect to cite 20–30 references that are most pertinent to your chapter.

Update Your Outline Based on the Literature Search

Your first outline was developed from your existing knowledge and your initial goals for the chapter. Once you have done a complete literature search, go back through the outline and revise it as needed.

Your revised outline may include:

- Additional points identified in the literature
- Specific information to include under each heading
- Detailed information on which figures to include
- Additional references to cite

Confirm you have included the material that the editors require. If you were given information about the content of other chapters, check that your material does not overlap extensively and that any shared areas complement one another.

Tip: A picture is worth a thousand words. If you include figures, choose high-quality images that relay key information easily.

Divide Work among Co-Authors and Establish Firm Deadlines

If there are co-authors on the chapter, discuss who will be the **lead author** and establish plans for creating the chapter. For example, the lead author may draft the chapter, then send it to the others to revise. Alternatively, each co-author may be assigned a section. The lead author would then revise the entire document to ensure the writing is consistent throughout.

Assign **responsibility for figures**. Decide who will obtain any permissions needed for copyrighted work, who will be responsible for any illustrations, and who will ensure all figures are formatted properly.

Establish **firm deadlines** for drafts to be completed. Indicate the allotted time for revisions to be made and set a date for all co-authors to turn in their final comments and revisions. The lead author should check in with co-authors regularly to make sure things are progressing according to schedule.

Note: The final chapter must be written with a **single voice**. It should never be apparent to the readers that different co-authors wrote different sections.

Tip: **Set the deadlines earlier than the editors' deadline** to ensure you have enough time to make necessary corrections to text and figures.

Hint: Work with reliable co-authors who will produce good work in a timely fashion.

WRITE FOR THE TARGET AUDIENCE

Like other forms of medical science writing, you will use clear and concise language to help others easily process the material. However, unlike other forms of medical science writing, you add a more personalized style to a book chapter. You can write as the expert that you are, providing opinions, anecdotes from your own experiences, and summaries and interpretations of previous work. You can use your knowledge to shape how others view the topic and share your thoughts about future priorities in the field. Of course, you must provide a balanced overview of the topic. For example, when you summarize your work, include information on what others have found, including any contradictory findings or interpretations.

How you convey your knowledge will depend on the book's purpose and target audience. For example, the writing styles used to describe orthopedic surgical procedures in a patient information guide, a college anatomy textbook, and a surgical manual for hand surgeons will be very different. **Even as the expert, you must adapt your writing style to fit the readers' needs**.

For many experts, adjusting their writing for a general audience is especially difficult. As an experienced clinician or researcher, you are used to talking about your work in certain terms. You are comfortable using words and abbreviations that are unfamiliar to other specialists. You are such an expert that you may not recognize that some words or descriptions may confuse readers.

To **make sure your writing is appropriate for the book's target audience**, have others read a draft of your chapter before you send it to the editor. To get the most useful feedback, **identify readers who are representative of the target audience**.

In addition to the writing style, **choose figures that help readers to understand** what you describe. **Consider** additional resources such as links to **videos** that demonstrate any concepts that are difficult to visualize. There are many online resources for experimental, clinical, and surgical techniques (**Box 14.4**).

Tip: If you struggle to explain complex information to a general audience, enlist a co-author from a different subfield or one with less experience. They can often identify sections that are too dense for non-experts to decipher.

> **Box 14.4   Faculty Perspective: Incorporating Links to Video Technology**
>
> While the training of surgical residents still requires direct mentoring in the operating room by a senior surgeon, current surgical residents often watch videos of the surgical procedures for which they are training. Many rely on content found online. A detailed discussion of the relevance of video technology is beyond the scope of this chapter; however, consider listing links to relevant online videos for any chapter in which surgical treatment is important. This technology provides the author with the opportunity to direct the readers to what the author considers to be the most relevant, up-to-date, surgical technology.
>
> Most subspecialty societies have libraries with video technology to support both current, innovative, new technologies, as well as older, tried-and-true procedures. For example, the American Society for Surgery of the Hand offers video links to "Hand-e" with hundreds of surgical videos. However, the videos are only available to members and candidate members. Authors should consider accessibility to the videos and include open access options as well.

14.4 CONCLUSIONS

Writing a book chapter provides opportunities to discuss your perspectives and opinions, and to shape the future of your field. The writing style is often more personalized and experience-based, giving authors an opportunity to share their ideas outside of the traditional journal format. Whenever you are invited to write a chapter, review the requirements and deadlines before committing to the project. If you are interested in the project, but concerned about the time commitment, recruit a reliable co-author to assist.

Although book chapters are usually not ranked as highly as peer-reviewed research publications for decisions regarding tenure and promotion, they remain important ways to make valuable scholarly contributions to one's field and are usually a rewarding experience for the authors.

REFERENCES AND RESOURCES

BOOKS
Scott-Conner C. *Medical Writing: Textbooks and Chapters.* Iowa City, IA: CreateSpace Independent Publishing; 2017.

ARTICLES
Kendirci M. How to write a medical book chapter? *Turk J Urol.* 2013;39(Suppl 1):37–40.
Mota P, Carvalho N, Carvalho-Dias E, et al. Video-based surgical learning: Improving trainee education and preparation for surgery. *J Surg Educ.* 2018;75(3):828–835.

CHAPTER 15

Attending and Presenting at Scientific Conferences: Common Elements

Alice Wang, M.D., Dominik Greda, M.D., Lynne M. Bianchi, Ph.D., and Calhoun D. Cunningham III, M.D.

Tips for Success:

> When you have a well-designed study with interesting preliminary data, share it with others.
>
> You do not need a study eligible for a top-ranking medical journal to present at a conference.

Warning:

> You will need to pare down your study description and results to fit conference presentation formats.

Key Concept: Conferences are a great way to disseminate your research findings, get valuable feedback, learn about others' work, and meet new colleagues.

As mentioned in Chapter 1, part of the research process is to disseminate your research findings. Sharing your study outcomes at a conference is one way to do that.

Many investigators present their work at a conference **poster session**. For these talks, a poster outlining the study purpose, results, and their meaning is displayed alongside other posters from other investigators. The posters are usually set up for several hours and investigators are assigned a specific time to be at their poster to discuss the study one-on-one with those who are interested. Other investigators speak at an **oral presentation**, also known as a podium talk. For this format, speakers create slides to explain their studies and results. Oral presentations are usually moderated, with speakers allotted 10–20 minutes to explain their research findings and answer questions from the audience. Oral presentations are usually held in large rooms so several attendees can hear the talk at one time. There are **similarities in the two forms of presentation**, such as the need to focus the presentation on the main findings, **as well as distinct elements**, such as how the content is organized and displayed.

DOI: 10.1201/9781003126478-15

You will likely attend many conferences throughout your career. These are valuable experiences, and you should prepare properly to make the most of each opportunity. In this chapter we provide an overview of common medical and science conference formats. Advice on how to prepare effective poster presentations (Chapter 16) and oral presentations (Chapter 17) follow.

Note: Presenting at conferences reflects favorably upon you, assuming you follow the conference guidelines and act professionally. Your presentations tell others that you follow projects through to completion, are organized, and motivated to share your ideas and results.

15.1 UNDERSTAND THE GOALS AND PURPOSES OF DIFFERENT PROGRAM FORMATS

There are multiple conference formats, ranging from small institutional gatherings to large national or international events. Some conferences showcase research by a group of students, residents, fellows, or other trainees at an institution. Others are organized by professional societies to highlight current practices, new discoveries, and innovations in the field(s) represented by that society. Some conferences focus on basic science, some on clinical work, and some include both. It is helpful to understand the characteristics of any conference you attend so you are prepared to make the most of each experience.

CONFERENCES

Academic conferences are the most common format for presenting new research and learning about new discoveries in your field of interest. These include small institutional conferences and large society meetings. Participants may include students, residents, other trainees, faculty, private practitioners, administrators, and industry representatives across multiple disciplines. Conferences typically have several educational formats, including keynote addresses, oral sessions, panel discussions, poster sessions, and, more recently, video sessions for surgical specialties.

Local conferences are organized by individuals at a single institution, or a few institutions located in the same geographic area. Faculty, administrators, and trainees may be involved in planning and organizing these conferences. Local conferences are often designed to highlight work conducted at the institution(s) and provide opportunities for students and trainees to present findings from their projects. These conferences may include poster and podium talks or only poster presentations. These are often one- or two-day events that may include keynote speakers. Because most attendees are from your institution you will likely know many of the people who view your work.

Some local conferences are organized solely to **showcase trainee work**. Some will allow residents to present updates to ongoing projects, while others only permit presentations summarizing completed projects. There may be judges who evaluate the posters or talks, and award prizes for the best presentations. **Judging criteria** are often focused on the organization and delivery of the presentation more than the actual outcomes of the study.

Local conferences are a great way to receive feedback on your project and presentation skills before presenting at a regional or national conference.

Note: Local conferences provide valuable practice before speaking at larger conferences. Residents often begin by presenting at small local conferences and then **share the same data** at a regional or national conference, **if permitted by conference guidelines**.

Tip: Residents and faculty should take advantage of opportunities to present at **local conferences**. These presentations **count as a scholarly activity** that is added to your *curriculum vitae* and the annual institutional scholarship reports. **Faculty mentors** should aim to co-author at least one resident presentation **annually** to demonstrate ongoing scholarly activity.

Hint: Be cautious of listing the same project title multiple times on your *curriculum vitae*. Make it obvious that the presentations differed in some way.

Warning: Although presentations at a local conference are usually accepted for submission at a larger conference, be aware that many national and international conferences stipulate that a project cannot have been previously presented at another national or international conference. Always check and adhere to submission guidelines.

Regional conferences are often organized by individuals at several different institutions, a subgroup of a professional society, or a state organization. Regional conferences may include keynote speakers, panel discussions, and podium and poster presentations. These conferences provide opportunities to get **feedback from others outside your institution**. You will meet others with similar interests and may develop collaborations with colleagues in your region. Like local conferences, many regional conferences award prizes to trainees.

National conferences are usually organized by professional societies or academies, and include attendees from across the country and sometimes from abroad. These conferences focus on topics related to the fields represented by the professional organization and include a mix of keynote speakers, panel discussions, seminars, podium talks, and poster presentations. Some national conferences attract thousands of attendees, whereas others, often targeted at a subspecialty, attract several hundred. National conferences provide great **learning and networking opportunities** as you will likely meet other trainees, established investigators, and leaders in your field.

National conferences, especially the larger ones, have multiple **concurrent sessions**, each focused on a different topic. This allows attendees to focus on the sessions of most interest to them. Podium sessions are often running at the same time as poster sessions and some attendees will go to portions of each to hear about specific studies of interest to them. Local and regional conferences may also run concurrent sessions, though for smaller conferences there may be no need to do so.

Some national conferences set aside time for trainees to present and may have judges and awards, whereas others have trainees mixed in with other presenters and do not offer prizes.

International conferences bring together experts from around the world and have many of the same formats and benefits as national conferences. International conferences provide opportunities to learn about medical research and treatments in other countries and can prove valuable to your development as a clinician and researcher. The costs associated with international travel may limit opportunities to attend these, particularly as a resident.

Note: Many national and international conferences offer **travel awards** to **trainees or junior faculty** to cover travel expenses. These are not only financially beneficial but are a recognized professional honor to be listed on your *curriculum vitae*. Be sure to explore these opportunities whenever you are eligible.

Tip: Several national and international medical conferences will publish your abstract in their associated journal. Some journals may require you to submit a full manuscript prior to the conference, providing another form of scholarly activity. Most require that the presented data were not previously published, so check requirements prior to submission.

Hint: **Look at the conference program ahead of time to make the most of concurrent sessions**. Each podium session lists the title, authors, and the time of each talk so attendees can choose those they want to hear. Sometimes, the entire session will be of interest to you; at other times, only a few talks will seem relevant. Each poster session lists the title, authors, and time at which the authors will be at their posters. The posters stay up for several hours and you can view the posters at any time during that session. For those posters of most interest to you, you can arrange to go when the authors are present.

OTHER TYPES OF SCIENTIFIC MEETINGS

Symposiums are typically smaller-scale academic conferences with a narrow focus. They attract experts in a particular field who meet to share their research findings regarding a specific topic and often make recommendations regarding a future course of action, such as revising patient care guidelines, recommending new curricular content, or summarizing topics in need of further research.

Seminars are educational events held by an academic institution or professional organization whereby one or more experts provide instruction or describe research regarding a particular topic. Academic departments frequently invite guest speakers and host seminars targeted at students, residents, and faculty.

Workshops usually represent an educational event with interactive participation by attendees. These meeting are typically moderated by an expert in the subject matter being discussed.

Conference webinars are internet-based conferences. The development of software platforms for virtual streaming provides increased opportunities to organize conferences on a national and international level. Benefits of this format include the ability to reach participants across a diverse geographic area, to reduce meeting and travel costs, and to provide on-demand access to presentations. Though missing the collegial aspect of socializing with fellow attendees, virtual meetings and conferences are a valuable format to disseminate scientific research.

15.2 FIT YOUR ABSTRACT AND PRESENTATION TO THE CONFERENCE

Both conference organizers and attendees want a conference that showcases high-quality work worthy of their time. To make a conference successful, organizers must address numerous logistics, such as booking spaces to house the conference and reserving accommodations for out-of-town attendees. Some organizers work with vendors who display equipment, devices, medications, books, or journals of interest to attendees. Organizers also assign speakers to the various podium or poster sessions.

As a meeting attendee, you do not need to know how to reserve a convention center, arrange for a block of rooms at a hotel, or vet vendors. What you should understand is that, for any conference, several **people volunteer many, many hours of time to make the conference flow smoothly**. Most conference organizers do not receive extra pay or time off for the work they do. As an attendee, appreciate the time that others devote to creating the event and **prepare an abstract and presentation that reflects positively on the conference**.

UNDERSTAND HOW CONFERENCE ABSTRACTS ARE REVIEWED AND ASSIGNED

Presenting at a conference typically begins with notification of a "call for abstracts." At this time, you **submit an abstract of your work**, usually several months in advance of the conference, to provide organizers with the time needed to review and schedule each presentation. Organizers look for abstracts that fit together in some way, often by topic, so attendees can focus on those presentations of most relevance to their interests. At local conferences and some regional conferences, sessions may be divided by type of presentation, department, trainee level, or some other criterion, rather than topic.

As discussed in Chapter 11, an abstract is a brief overview of a study that conveys essential information in only a few hundred words, or less. The introduction, methods, results, and discussion are presented in enough detail for others to understand what the study is about before coming to your presentation. **The abstract is often the only record attendees have of your presentation, so it needs to be clear, informative, and accurate**.

Consider the purpose and goals of the conference to make sure your project is a good fit. Write your abstract so it is clear why your study will be of interest to attendees.

Follow all instructions. Every conference dictates the **format**, **font size**, and **word or character limit** for abstract submissions. Those that do not meet criteria are usually not considered.

Check that the authors meet the eligibility criteria. Some conferences accept submissions from students, residents, and fellows, others only accept abstracts co-authored by senior faculty or members of the sponsoring society.

Note the abstract review criteria. Some conferences have strict review criteria and only accept a subset of the abstracts submitted, whereas others accept all abstracts that meet formatting and topic criteria. No matter what the criteria for abstract acceptance, write an abstract that reflects positively on you and your work.

Note presentation options. Some conferences allow you to **choose** whether you will present an oral or poster presentation, while others **assign** you to one or the other based on the topic of your presentation and the needs of the conference. Presentation options may differ for faculty and students/residents/fellows. For many medical conferences, being selected to give an oral presentation is an honor.

Write a helpful abstract. Explain your work in terms that are understood by those outside your area of expertise and provide enough detail about your findings so organizers are confident you will have something to present. Although many studies described at conferences are works in progress, projects should be sufficiently developed so there is something worthwhile to share (**Box 15.1**). It reflects poorly on the conference if there are presentations without substantial content.

Keep the perspective of the organizers in mind. Like you, conference organizers are busy with clinical work, research, and other duties. To make the review process easier for them, prepare a clearly written abstract, following all guidelines. Make sure the abstract is understood by those outside your area of expertise and is easy to assign to a session. Get feedback from a colleague not associated with the project to make sure you have written it in an accessible manner.

Tip: Before submitting your abstract, confirm you have adhered to the word or character limit and formatted the abstract as required for that conference.

Hint: Make sure the title and content of the abstract match so organizers are not confused about where your work fits.

Note: Sometimes, presenters are surprised when they are assigned to a session that does not fit their research topic and they blame the organizers for not paying attention. However, if a presentation is placed in an inappropriate group, it is often due to lack of clarity in the submitted abstract.

Box 15.1   When Things Go Wrong

You wrote an abstract describing your preliminary results and it was accepted for a talk at a national conference. The preliminary data were interesting, but you needed to gather more data, which you noted in your abstract. However, after you collect the additional data, you discover there are problems. Perhaps now that you have a larger sample size you discover there is no difference between the experimental and control groups as you reported in your abstract. Perhaps you discover an inaccuracy with the measurement tool or problems with your control conditions. Now what do you do?

Sometimes, preliminary data are misleading. Sometimes, data collection is flawed. These things happen. One option is to withdraw your abstract. If you discover a major flaw and there is nothing worth presenting, that may be the best option. However, conferences are a place where people present studies in progress so having incomplete data or data different from the abstract is not unusual. You may be able to present what happened, explain what you found, and describe what you will do next. It is okay to state that preliminary data suggested differences, but with a larger sample size you found there were no differences. The lack of a difference still tells you something. You may be able to explain what was wrong with the measurement tool and what revisions you made to correct it. That too provides information to others who may be interested in doing a similar study. You want to present what you found, even if it is not what you planned to discuss. Use the presentation as an opportunity to share your experience with others.

Discuss with your mentor and co-authors the best way to deal with any issues that arise after abstract submission.

Note: Although the unexpected may happen after you submit an abstract, **do not write your abstract in a way that promises data you do not have**. If the project is at such an early stage that you do not have clear results, it is better to wait until you collect enough valid data before submitting an abstract to a conference.

TARGET YOUR ABSTRACT AND PRESENTATION TO A BROAD AUDIENCE

Those who attend conferences represent individuals at every career stage. Some attendees will be leaders in the field who were invited to give keynote speeches. Others are mid-career professionals with long-standing research programs, who use conferences to discuss their latest findings. Others are new investigators presenting some of their early research, and some are trainees presenting for the very first time.

It is helpful to keep in mind the **diverse nature of participants** when developing your abstract and presentation. You want your abstract to be easily understood so people become interested in attending your presentation. When presenting, you want your information to be as accessible to a student attending his first conference as it is to an experienced investigator interested in the details of your techniques. **Pitching a presentation to a broad audience is always a challenge**, but with **planning** and **rehearsal** you can **develop a presentation that meets the needs of different attendees**.

The chapters that follow explain how to prepare for oral and poster presentations. Whether explaining your data using slides or a poster board, you need to condense your project goals and results into a succinct presentation that is easy to follow. Slides and posters need to be easy to read from a distance, eye-catching, but not distracting. Your "take-home message," the main point you want the audience to remember from your presentation, needs to be obvious. Your choice of **words, text size, colors,** and **graphics** all **impact how well an audience processes your content**.

How you present influences how well attendees understand your project. **You will need to practice your talk, whether you are giving it at a podium or a poster**, so that you clearly and concisely explain to the audience what you did and what you found.

PREPARE AN UNBIASED ABSTRACT AND PRESENTATION

As you prepare your abstract and presentation, it is helpful to remember that the data you collect are not a reflection of your intelligence. How you set up and report the results are what reflect your abilities. Too often, investigators view a hypothesis as right/wrong, good/bad. Some seem to think that, if the data support the hypothesis, the project is good, and the investigator is smart. In contrast, if the data do not support the study objectives, the project is bad, and the investigator is not smart. Science is about finding information; data that do not support a hypothesis still provide information.

When presenting your work, **state your hypothesis and results without emotional attachment and without overstating findings**. You are presenting data, not your opinions on the outcomes. Use concise, simple sentences, avoiding excessive adjectives and "flowery" descriptions. Avoid words like "hope," "disappointed," or "pleased." Avoid stating that values are higher or lower if there is no statistically significant difference. There is no need to say anything about data being "almost significant" or "trending toward significant." Others will find that misleading, at best. If your results are not statistically significant, say so and provide your statistical outcomes for viewers to see.

Examples:

> Use: "We hypothesized …"
> Avoid: "We *hoped* to show …"

> Use: "There were no differences between groups"
> Avoid: "*Unfortunately*, there were no differences between groups."

> Use: "Mean scores were similar for the low-dose and mid-dose groups."
> Avoid: "The mean score for the low-dose group was *higher* than that for the mid-dose group, *but* the difference was *not statistically significant*."

Remember: The data are not a reflection on your intelligence; however, your ability to carry out a well-controlled study and present it clearly and accurately are.

Note: As a resident, you may present your research only at a local conference. You may view such presentations as unimportant experiences. However, **the process of preparing and presenting your research is quite valuable**, as you will likely attend and present at other conferences in your career. The training and practice you receive as a resident will make subsequent presentations better.

Tip: As a resident, it is helpful to **gain experience giving both poster and oral presentations**. Many people prefer posters because they allow for direct interaction with others and do not seem as stress-inducing as standing at a podium before a large audience. However, both formats have advantages, and residency is a good time to try both. Fortunately, **audiences are generally empathetic to new investigators**, and being nervous or stumbling over some words are forgivable offenses.

Hint: At many regional and national conferences, the projects thought to be most impactful are assigned as oral presentations as these generally reach a larger audience than poster presentations. Although potentially more stressful for many speakers, oral presentations are a welcome assignment.

15.3 USE CONFERENCES TO BUILD YOUR PROFESSIONAL NETWORK

Presenting at a conference is one of the best ways to network with others in your field. Presenting your work not only demonstrates your research accomplishments, but gives others insight into your interests, critical thinking, and organizational and communication skills. The connections you make at conferences often lead to new collaborations and the identification of colleagues qualified to serve as reviewers for your manuscripts and grants.

Those who attend conferences on a regular basis often find themselves getting together with the same groups of people each year. The **social side of a conference** is sometimes overlooked, but it is one of the greatest benefits to attending. The colleagues you meet may become future mentors or co-workers. As a resident, you may meet someone who later hires you to work in their department. **Many job opportunities, research collaborations**, and **lifelong friendships begin at conferences**.

Socializing is an important part of any conference but pay attention to how you present yourself (Box 15.2). For example, it is not unusual for a group to get together at the end of the day to discuss work over a beer or other alcoholic beverage. In some fields, such gatherings are considered the norm. However, there is an **important distinction between discussing work over a drink and drinking**. If you choose to drink with colleagues, due so with caution and maintain your professional standards. Some careers are helped by a conversation over a beer, some are hurt, usually because there is more than one drink imbibed. Of course, if you do not usually drink alcohol, a conference would not be the place to start.

Box 15.2   Blending the Work and Social Aspects of Conferences

National conferences are held in cities large enough to accommodate the influx of several hundred to several thousand attendees and are often organized in desirable geographic locations with interesting attractions. Conference organizers often point out local attractions and attendees may set aside time to tour the region. Dining at local restaurants and taking in sites are common and positive aspects of conference attendance. It is important, however, to balance the time you spend at the conference with any time you spend sightseeing.

Some attendees bring family members with them to create a sort of "working vacation." However, it is important to think about how you will use your time at the meeting and the pros and cons of mixing family travel with a conference. One of the major benefits of attending larger conferences is the opportunity to meet new colleagues. If you are dividing your day between vacationing and conferencing, you will likely miss some talks you should attend, and your decreased presence will limit networking opportunities. If you must rush back at the end of the day to meet family, you may miss out on opportunities to talk with others over dinner. If you decline invitations due to family obligations, others may sense you are not dedicated to your work or interested in theirs. **Arranging for family to arrive and depart either before or after the meeting is one way to minimize distractions**.

You should always **check with your institution regarding policies and procedures for family travel** to conference locations and how to separate your eligible travel expenses for reimbursement.

15.4 CONCLUSIONS

Attending and presenting at a scientific meeting provides a stimulating opportunity to connect with colleagues in your field, meet new people, stay up-to-date on current advances, and gain valuable feedback regarding your work. Although often packed with a tremendous educational curriculum, conferences also promote both professional and social connections. Whether you decide to pursue an academic or clinical career, the opportunity to present at a conference is a rewarding experience that will likely provide further self-improvement, enhance your intellectual curiosity, and expand your network of colleagues.

REFERENCES AND RESOURCES

BOOK
Lang TA. *How to Write, Publish, and Present in the Health Sciences: A Guide for Clinicians and Laboratory Researchers*. Philadelphia: American College of Physicians; 2010.

ARTICLES
Jasko JJ, Wood JH, Schwartz HS. Publication rates of abstracts presented at annual musculoskeletal tumor society meetings. *Clin Orthop Relat Res*. 2003;415:98–103.

Mata H, Latham TP, Ransome Y. Benefits of professional organization membership and participation in national conferences: Considerations for students and new professionals. *Health Promot Pract*. 2010;11(4):450–453.

Thomas M, Inniss-Richter Z, Mata H, Cottrell RR. Career development through local chapter involvement: Perspectives from chapter members. *Health Promot Pract*. 2013;14(4):480–484

Zierath JR. Building bridges through scientific conferences. *Cell* 2016;167(5):1155–1158.

See also references and resources specific to poster presentations (Chapter 16) and oral presentations (Chapter 17).

Preparing and Giving Effective Poster Presentations

Alice Wang, M.D., Dominik Greda, M.D., Sean Carroll, D.O.,
Lynne M. Bianchi, Ph.D., and Calhoun D. Cunningham III, M.D.

Tips for Success:

> *Plan your poster around two or three key points.*
> *Organize the content so your results and significance are easy to comprehend.*

Warning:

> *Failure to prepare and present a poster at the appropriate level reflects*
> *poorly on you, your co-authors, and your institution.*

Key Concept: Posters are an important form of scholarly activity.

Poster presentations are an important means of succinctly presenting research findings and, not surprisingly, poster sessions are found at nearly every medical and science conference. At first, a poster presentation may seem like a casual event or might remind you of a grade school science fair. However, **poster presentations** are an established form of scholarship and always should be treated as **important and influential scholarly activities**. Presenting a poster allows you to discuss your work one-on-one with other attendees and often leads to further collaborative and collegial opportunities.

As a busy resident focused on completing graduation requirements and applying for the next fellowship or job, you might not rank poster presentations high on your priority list. That would be a mistake. **The quality of your poster, even more than the data itself, leaves an impression on others**. You want to make sure that the impression is a favorable one. This chapter provides tips on how to organize and present a poster that effectively shares your findings with other conference attendees.

Note: Some residents present results of a small study at a local conference that highlights resident research. The temptation to throw something together at the last minute may be great. Avoid that temptation. The **final product you create will leave an impression on those at your residency institution**. You never know who will wander by and see your poster. Administrators, physicians in other departments, various health care providers, fellow residents, students, and others may view your poster. **Do not**

DOI: 10.1201/9781003126478-16

provide an opportunity for others to think you are careless, uninterested, or lazy. You have all of residency to demonstrate those traits, should you wish.

16.1 RECOGNIZE THE ELEMENTS OF A SUCCESSFUL POSTER: FOCUS AND CLARITY

There are many resources with advice on how to prepare and present an effective poster. The advice is largely the same: **keep your poster focused, limit the text, guide your reader to quickly understand the key points**. Yet, despite all the sage advice and numerous examples available, every conference has several posters that look like they were selected to provide examples of what *not* to do.

The first thing to note is that your poster is *not* a "manuscript on board." You must deliberately choose what text and images to include and how and where to place each item. The information should tell a story. It should be concise and presented in a "bullet-point" fashion where appropriate, so readers can quickly grasp the purpose and findings of your study.

As with other forms of writing, **keep your audience in mind** when preparing a poster. Your audience will be attendees with diverse backgrounds. Like you, each will attend multiple posters and learn about a variety of studies. Like you, other attendees want to process as much information as they can in the time available. Thus, it is essential to provide information that is **clear**, **concise**, and **easily processed**.

Note: Although you must be selective in what you present, you **cannot omit negative results** or **exclude conflicting data** simply because they do not support your study objectives. It is acceptable and wise to limit your poster to main findings, but it is not acceptable or ethical to select only the results that support your hypothesis. Your goal is to present a clear overview of what you found. If what you found is inconsistent with your study objectives, you include those results.

Tip: Design your poster for the tired, overstimulated attendee.

Hint: At many conferences, **prizes are awarded** for the best posters. Such awards are an honor worth putting on your *curriculum vitae*. Do not underestimate the importance of creating an appealing, concise, and informative poster to represent your work.

PLAN THE POSTER LAYOUT: KEY POINTS TO CONSIDER

Less Is More

Include only the essential information. For each poster section, ask, "What are the most important things for readers to know?" Choose a few key points that you would like attendees to remember and build your poster around those.

Organize in Chunks

There are many effective layouts for organizing a poster, such as the format shown in Figure 16.1. Whatever format you choose, be sure to arrange the

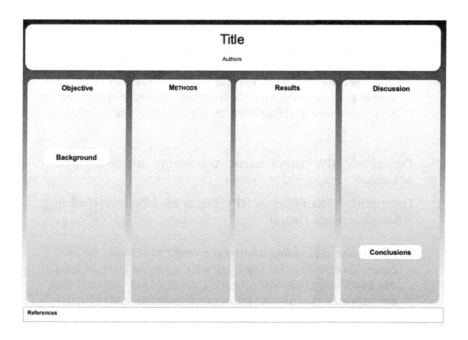

Figure 16.1 An example of a poster layout with content organized in chunks. Headings and organization will differ based on conference guidelines and author preference. For example, the abstract may be included in place of, or in addition to, the "Objective."

content so the **essential information** is easily seen by those walking past. Viewers should be able to **see the main points easily from ten feet away**.

To make it easier for viewers to process information, leave **space between sections** and make **headings a larger font than the main text**. Some readers will seek out the results or conclusions first, so make it easy for them to quickly locate these sections as they pass by your poster.

Balance Information and Visual Appeal

Provide a **layout that attracts others to your poster**. Envision thirty people walking down a row of posters trying to choose one to read. Typically, a person will first notice the aesthetics of your poster, then the title. To get others interested in your poster, make it easy to find information and quickly gather key points.

> *Use a text size large enough to read from a distance.* Unless otherwise instructed by conference guidelines, text font should be at **minimum 28-point font**. Headings should be kept at 34 to 36-point font. The easier it is to read, the more likely people will pay attention.

> *Make and place images, graphs, tables, and photos that are easily viewed from a distance.* Consider both the size and location of all the

content. One may need to get closer to examine the details of a microscopic image or a patient scan, but it should be obvious to those walking past what the images are displaying.

Compose a declarative title that highlights the main result of your study. Rather than describe what the study was about, inform the reader what you found. Declarative titles tend to attract more readers.

Examples:

Declarative: "HPV Status Predicts 5-Year Survival in Oropharyngeal Cancer."

Descriptive: "The Effect of HPV Status on 5-Year Survival in Oropharyngeal Cancer."

Put a concise subheading above each result to indicate the outcome. Make it easy for someone walking by to learn at least one key finding from your poster. Even if they do not read the entire poster, they should know one thing your study found.

Examples:

"Genetically modified neurons did not adhere to a laminin substrate."

"Cookie consumption decreased subjective pain scores in children."

Tip: **Your poster should be visually appealing but not "flashy."** The goal is to draw the readers' attention to key points. Too much color, ornate designs, or other distracting features, no matter how artistic, will dissuade people from stopping at your poster. A flashy poster may give some the impression that you are not a serious scientist and others the feeling that you are compensating for a lack of interesting data.

Hint: **Text-heavy** posters are **ignored** by attendees. Try to **replace text** with **clear figures** to support your key results. Easy-to-follow posters are considered good, even by those who do not read them.

Remember: When selecting colors, consider that **many people are colorblind** and **adjust your final design** to make your findings **easily read** by different viewers. There are many different color combinations that viewers have difficulty distinguishing. To make your poster appealing to the widest readership, be sure to check the contrast in each section and choose a color scheme that does not cause eye strain. If you have color images, it is helpful to look at your final poster in gray scale to see if your main findings still stand out as you expect. In addition to using colors, where possible, use additional features such as icons, arrows, or pictographs to get your point across.

INCLUDE THE EXPECTED CONTENT IN EACH SECTION

In general, posters follow the **same format as a manuscript**, but with **much less detail** in each section. Except for case reports and case series (**Box 16.1**), most posters at medical and science conferences follow the IMRaD format (Introduction, Methods, Results, and Discussion), though different headings may be preferred (e.g., Background in place of Introduction, Summary instead of Discussion).

Although your poster is arranged in a standard format, many who stop at your poster will read the sections out of order. Some attendees will first scan the abstract to see what the study is about; others will start by reading the conclusions. Some will look at the figures first. Because you will not know where a viewer will start reading, **each section should stand alone and highlight a "take-home message."**

Abstract: A Brief Overview of the Study and Your Findings

You typically submit an abstract in advance of the conference, as explained in Chapter 15. You usually include a copy of this abstract at the beginning of your poster. You do not re-write your abstract for the poster and in general should not make any changes to the abstract, other than to correct typographical errors.

If there are substantial differences in what your abstract indicated based on additional data you collected after submission, you might highlight the changes in italics or at the end of the abstract to alert readers there are differences from the abstract printed in the program.

If helpful, and conference guidelines allow, you can make the text a little smaller than the rest of the poster since the same information is in the conference abstract book available to attendees. However, do not make it so small no one can read it from a distance. Not everyone reads or recalls the abstracts printed in a program.

Always consult your conference guidelines to see if there are restrictions on content changes or text size.

Introduction: Why Was the Study Done; Why Is It Interesting?

The introduction should highlight **why your study was needed**. Briefly describe what was previously known about your topic and what required investigation. Write the introduction so readers quickly understand the **purpose and importance** of your study. Generally, the introduction will not extend past the first column of the poster.

You will include some **references** to alert the reader to other work in the field, but a poster does not include a full literature review. Cite only references directly relevant to your presentation and use review articles, if available. However, be familiar with the broader literature and be prepared to discuss other studies with those who come to your poster.

Tip: **Lists of key points are often easier to read than full paragraphs.**

Hint: The goal is to get your points across clearly and easily. **Experiment with layouts** that use lists, bullet points, or underlining and bolded text to convey important information.

Remember: Write your introduction so readers are curious to see what happened in your study. You do *not* need to have a paradigm-shifting discovery for your study to be interesting. Smaller contributions are important too. Readers simply need to understand how your study adds something to the field.

Methods: How Was the Study Done?

This is one section where more text is expected and acceptable, within reason. Consider what information is needed to understand how the study was conducted. What a reader needs to know about a project using immunohistochemical techniques is quite different from what one needs to know about a study using an investigator-created patient survey.

You typically indicate the **study design, sample size, control conditions** and any **statistical analyses** you used. For methods commonly used, you can state, "In brief…" followed by a short overview and appropriate citations. Details of any modifications to those methods should be included.

As with every section of the poster, organize the information to make comprehension as easy as possible. You might list steps or create a flow chart or other diagram to help readers follow your approach.

Hint: **This section should *not* be the longest one on your poster.** Keep the methods focused on the key elements required to understand how the study was completed. Attendees can discuss your methods in more detail if they are interested.

Results: What Were the Main Findings?

The **results section** of the poster is of **primary interest to most viewers,** so you want to make it as informative and visually appealing as possible.

Include **figures,** such as **images, graphs, tables,** and **illustrations** to highlight and summarize your findings easily. **Experiment** with the **layout, sizes,** and **colors** to find what works best. For example, note whether data are better presented in a graph or a table.

Consider how the order of presentation impacts comprehension. In some cases, you may find the best organization for presenting the results is different from the order in which the data were gathered.

A **succinct subheading** should be placed above each figure to inform readers of the main finding. For example, "Aerobic exercise increased acne in adults" would be placed above the figure and text detailing this result. Together, the subheadings should convey all the important findings of your study. Prepare subheadings so attendees who only read these know what your study found.

Place figures at a location and height that is easily viewed. Avoid putting images in areas that are clearly above or below eye level for most attendees (see **Box 16.2**). **Figure legends** should be brief yet detailed enough to let readers know what they are viewing. To improve clarity, imagine readers do not have access to the rest of the poster.

Make any labels, arrows, color differences, or icons easy to spot. A frustrated viewer is likely to move on to the next poster.

Note: Keep the available space and primary story in mind when deciding what to include. Secondary findings can be discussed at the poster or briefly summarized in a single paragraph without figures, if appropriate.

Tip: There should be no "surprises" hidden in the text of the poster. Those who skim the poster, those who read only the headings and subheadings, and those who read the poster in its entirety should all walk away knowing what your study found.

Hint: Of all the sections of the poster, the **results** section is the one you are likely to reorganize and revise the most. You revise all poster sections multiple times, but this section will take more time to **create an eye-catching, easily digested format**.

Remember: **Not all results need to be on the poster**. You often have more data than you can include in a single poster, particularly if you have a study with more than one aim or multiple outcomes.

Discussion: What Do the Findings Mean? What Needs to Be Done Next?

This section interprets your findings, explains how they relate to other work, and indicates work which remains to be done.

Highlight the meaning of each key finding using **short paragraphs (2–4 sentences)** or **a list of summary points**. Put spaces between the findings so viewers can identify them easily.

Write your summary points so **anyone who reads this section first has a good understanding of what your study found**.

Examples:

> "Our genetically modified neurons failed to adhere to a laminin substrate because they lacked integrin receptors."

> "Children aged 7–10 were able to complete our patient satisfaction survey without prompts, whereas those aged 4–6 lacked the language skills to process the questions independently."

You may cite **references** in this section to indicate how your work relates to other work in the field. However, as with the introduction section of your poster, you are not trying to replicate the information included in a manuscript. Review articles can be cited, but you should be prepared to discuss other literature related to your study. You do not want to give the impression yours is the only study ever done in the area, yet you need to limit references to those directly related to your findings.

A statement highlighting **future directions** and **limitations** of the study should be included. This helps viewers know where you are going with the study or what other studies need to be done to clarify remaining issues.

You can combine the limitations with the future directions.

Examples:

> "Our results only include analysis of adults over age 75. Studies of adults aged 50–74 are currently in progress."

> "This study was limited to a small sample from a single location. Future work is needed to determine whether the results are generalizable to all patients with Parkinson's disease."

Conclusion: What Is the Take-Home Message? What Should Others Remember about Your Study?

A final statement is included at the end of the discussion or under a separate heading. This should be **one** or **two sentences** capturing what you most want readers to know about your study.

Examples:

> "We successfully created genetically modified neurons that lack integrin receptors."

> "A child-centered patient satisfaction survey was developed for outpatient services."

Tip: Imagine this is the only section a viewer reads on your poster.

Hint: Viewers may start by reading the discussion/summary/conclusions to see if they want to read the full poster. **Write these sections so they are clear,**

factual, and **interesting enough to entice someone to look at the rest of your poster**. However, do not "oversell" your results or make your findings appear more impressive than they are. You are a physician-scientist, and your poster should reflect your thoughtful and ethical work.

References: What Works Did You Cite in Your Poster?

Include all references cited in your poster. You can make this section a smaller font if allowed by conference guidelines, but not so small that it is difficult to read even when standing in front of it. Many attendees will not look at your references; however those who are most interested in your work will want to know what other papers you have read and may take notes. Therefore, **make sure your citations are accurate and complete**.

Box 16.1   Case Reports: Special Considerations

Many residents present findings from a case report. These too should be easy to follow with plenty of spaces to highlight relevant information. As with any poster, you must make **key points easy to find**. Include **only relevant images** and, if helpful, put patient information in a table to make it easier to digest quickly.

Keep your readers in mind and create a poster that one can process in about five minutes. You may think everything about your case report is important, but that is unlikely. Few people will stop to read a text-heavy report, no matter how fascinating the case.

As with other studies, you can fill in additional details when you discuss your findings with others. You cannot, however, discuss your findings with people who do not come to your poster, so avoid discouraging viewers with a poster densely packed with text and images.

16.2 PUT THE POSTER TOGETHER THOUGHTFULLY

In the past, posters were created on poster boards with text and figures printed out and pasted onto the boards. Now, most posters are printed as single large sheets, using computer software and available templates. Your institution may have a printing office or a contract with a local printer. You may be limited to a few templates, have several to choose from, or have the option to design your own layout. You may be encouraged to use institution colors and logos. Some printing offices provide the option of printing on paper or cloth. Cloth is more expensive, but easier to carry when traveling and particularly helpful for international travel.

If you do not have access to printed posters, **poster board** and paper still work well. You can print the text and most figures from your computer.

ORGANIZE THE LAYOUT ON PRINTED SHEETS OR POSTER BOARDS

Whatever options are available for creating your poster, **schedule enough time to experiment with the layout, colors, fonts, and spacing before the final printing**.

Even with templates, it takes time to develop an effective layout and to size figures appropriately. When using computer templates, use a grid to help align the elements of your poster.

If you are using poster board and paper, be prepared to spend more time than you anticipate necessary for printing and cutting (and re-printing and re-cutting) text and figures. Determine where each item will be placed before pasting any materials onto the board. Talk with others who have used this method to get advice on how best to attach the text and figures (glue, paste, or full-sheet printer labels) and how to cut the board to make it easier to carry.

Your **conference guidelines** usually have specifications for **poster sizes**. Make your poster as large as allowed so the font size, spacing, and image sizes are easier to read. However, do not make it larger than the recommended size or it will hang over the edges of the poster stands and be distracting, rather than inviting.

REVIEW YOUR POSTER AS IT MIGHT APPEAR TO SOMEONE ELSE
Once you have what you think is the final text and layout, evaluate your poster as if you did not already know the content. Did you write your poster so that it is **accessible to a broad audience**? Do headings and figure legends make sense if read in isolation?

Remember, you are not trying to impress the experts in the field by leaving out information you assume they know or to showcase your brilliance with excessive technical jargon. Even experts get tired after viewing several posters and, by the second day of a conference, most attendees are suffering from information overload. Check that you have written in a manner **easily comprehended** by others.

Is the **layout uncluttered *and* easy to follow**? Do you have a balance of text, empty space, and figures? Consider whether the colors complement one another and provide the contrast necessary for those readers who have difficulty distinguishing color combinations. Does your layout incorporate the advice in **Box 16.2** and **Box 16.3**?

Note: The easier your poster is to follow, the more impressed others will be with your work

Tip: A handy rule-of-thumb that many people use when designing a poster is that the **average person scans a poster in 10 seconds from 10 feet away**. It is also recommended that the **content be understandable within 10 minutes**, or less. Keep these recommendations in mind when creating your poster.

Hint: Review conference guidelines and required elements prior to printing the final poster.

Box 16.2   Spend Time Experimenting with the Layout

Imagine what your poster will look like once hung up in a row with 40 other posters around it. Will it stand out in a positive way? Then imagine yourself in front of the poster pointing things out to people. What do you want to highlight? What do viewers need to know?

Put main points where they will be most easily seen. You do not want a key image to be too high up for most viewers or in a lower corner where people must crouch over to see what you want them to observe. You do not want to discover at the conference that you have to stand on your toes and extend your arm high above your head to point to an essential part of a figure. Not everything can be ideally placed but be sure to put thought into what should be located most centrally and how you will point to important elements.

Spread the information out so that text-heavy areas are balanced with spaces and images. Avoid continuing paragraphs from one column or section to the next wherever possible. Break up your information into chunks and leave spaces between paragraphs and sections. This will make it easier for viewers to process and remind you what to emphasize as you present.

PROOFREAD

It may seem obvious that you will check the spelling, punctuation, and grammar carefully before printing your poster. Yet, typographical errors are very easy to overlook and the more familiar you are with a document, the harder it is to find them. It helps to set the poster aside for a day or two, then read it again.

After proofreading the poster carefully from the beginning, **read the sections out of sequence** (Summary, Results, Methods, Introduction, Abstract) and **read sentences backward**. Both methods help you pick up errors your brain would otherwise correct.

After you have corrected all the identified mistakes, have someone else read it over before you print the final version. It is very easy to miss your own mistakes, even when you carefully review each word.

Multiple typographical errors, misplaced headings or captions, or other glaring mistakes leave a negative impression. **People often remember mistakes more than the findings** so be sure to check over everything multiple times. A single typographical error is not a serious issue, but several mistakes, even small ones, give the **impression of carelessness or incompetence**.

16.3 PRESENT YOUR POSTER EFFECTIVELY

The tips used to create an effective and easy-to-follow layout also serve as a guide for your presentation. A poster is in some ways like a large cue card that reminds presenters what to say. However, unlike the cue cards used by speakers or actors, you do not read directly from the poster.

REHEARSE

Presenting a **poster** effectively **requires rehearsal**. You need to practice what you are going to say, just as you would for an oral presentation. You should have a **smooth** and **polished 5- to 7-minute overview** that you are prepared to present each time someone comes up to your poster.

You may think rehearsing is unnecessary because everything is already printed and organized, allowing you to simply follow the poster and read the text as you present. However, you will not have time to read your entire poster and viewers will not appreciate it if you do. **Attendees have many posters to view so keep your presentation clear, focused, and brief**. Those who wish to discuss your project further will ask questions and stay longer.

Failure to rehearse will result in awkward and uncomfortable interactions. The day of the conference is not the time to discover that you are unsure of how to explain the methods in less than two minutes or how to transition from one finding to the next. **Practice what you will say, what you will highlight, and where you will point on the poster**. Make your talk a bit different from the text on the poster so viewers feel you are talking with them and not reading to them.

At the conference, use your rehearsed talk as a starting point but **be prepared to go off-script**. Make eye contact with the viewers as you speak and stop periodically to see if they have questions. Treat the poster as the focus of a discussion between you and those who viewing it.

Some attendees may stand and look blankly at the poster as you describe your work and then just walk away. Some people are like that at a conference. One or two of those should not alarm you. However, if more people do that than not, you are probably not paying attention to the viewers in a way that invites conversation.

Remember: The **best presentations** and **most fruitful interactions occur when presenters rehearse before the meeting**. You may never give your talk exactly as rehearsed, but having thoughts clarified ahead of time will make for a better presentation.

CONVEY AN INVITING ATTITUDE WHEN STANDING AT THE POSTER

Most conferences assign a time for you to stand by your poster. The assigned time slot is often 30–90 minutes long. An assigned time lets other attendees know when to come by if they wish to speak with you. It also allows you unscheduled time to attend other presentations.

When you are at your poster, **stand to the side** waiting for people to approach; **do not** stand in the center and **block the poster**. When people come up to your poster, introduce yourself and offer to take them through your poster. Some viewers will decline, preferring to read the poster before deciding if they want to discuss anything with you. Others will indicate they want you to give them the overview. If so, begin your rehearsed talk.

Some investigators underestimate the importance of offering to present the poster. Too often a presenter stands by the poster and waits to see if someone asks a question. This is not a helpful approach and often causes people to wander off without discussing your work with you. **A poster presentation is a chance to talk with others in your field so make sure you convey an inviting attitude**. Discussions at a poster often provide additional insight into your project or suggestions on how to improve your study. The feedback you get at a poster is often helpful in preparing a subsequent manuscript for publication.

Consider having a handout, business cards, or even a quick response (QR) code on the poster. These additions help interested attendees remember your study and often facilitate future collaboration.

Tip: As a new investigator, you may not get as much "traffic" as some other presenters. **Encourage your friends and colleagues to stop by** so you can go through your rehearsed presentation with them. Other attendees are likely to hear parts of your talk, and some will become interested enough to stop and read your poster or ask questions. **However, do not have your friends stay and chat with you the entire time** as that discourages others from reading your poster and asking questions.

Hint: Conversations at a poster, including those unrelated to your poster, are overheard by other attendees.

ANTICIPATE QUESTIONS

Think about the many questions and issues that came up as you worked on your project and try to predict questions others are likely to ask. Consult co-authors and colleagues to identify additional questions that may arise. Once you have developed a list of questions and appropriate answers, **rehearse answering them** so that you have a polished response.

Once at the meeting, you will likely be asked other questions as well, including some you cannot answer. If possible, explain why you do not know. It may be as simple as, "We do not have enough data yet to answer that," or "Our methods cannot detect such differences." In other cases, you simply will not have an answer. Acknowledge when that is the case, and, if appropriate, indicate you will try to find the answer. You may also want to ask a follow-up question to see if the viewer has any experience or insight that might address the question asked.

Tip: Make sure you **listen to the questions** and **answer what is asked**. Sometimes, you will be expecting a question and have a rehearsed answer. If someone asks something similar, you may launch into your prepared answer without ever realizing you are not answering the question. Listen carefully to the full question before you begin your answer.

Hint: Ending your response with, "Did that address your question?" demonstrates your interest in the viewer and invites additional discussion.

Remember: **If you do not know the answer to something, admit it** rather than trying to make up something on the spot. Keep track of the questions you do not have answers for so you can address them later.

BE PREPARED FOR UNFRIENDLY ATTENDEES

Some people like to challenge every data point and interpretation. Some do so in an inquisitive manner, others in an offensive manner. You should **be prepared for rudeness** but **avoid being defensive**. Always consider what people are saying, rather than how they are saying it. Some points may be valid and help you improve your study. If the person has misunderstood something about your project or data, you can clarify the information.

Whether the comments are helpful or not, thank the person for stopping to discuss your work. It is important to avoid getting into a heated discussion or debate. Handling yourself well in the face of rudeness takes practice but reflects positively on you. Other nearby attendees will respect your composure and, every so often, the rudest attendee you encounter later becomes your greatest advocate because you handled yourself well under trying circumstances.

Remember: The better the presentation, the more impressed people will be, no matter what the results of the study. **Being professional, polished, thoughtful, and knowledgeable about your work are the keys to a successful poster presentation**.

DRESS FOR SUCCESS

Dress appropriately and professionally. Although the type of conference dictates the dress code, whatever the standards, look professional. Because poster presentations are considered less formal than oral presentations, many presenters dress less formally. At many conferences, presenters will be in "dress casual" clothing, such as slacks with polo shirts, button-down shirts, or blouses. Poster presenters at some medical conferences wear business-style clothing, such as a coat and tie, or skirt, dress, or slacks with a jacket. Always follow the norms of your conference and subfield, but never appear too casual.

Note: At some science conferences, jeans and T-shirts are common. However, as a physician, you should dress more professionally.

Tip: Some conferences are held in warm and sunny places that convey a vacation-like atmosphere. Avoid the temptation to wear shorts, sandals, or swimwear, even if you see others dressing that way.

Hint: You want others to remember your data, not your clothing, or lack of.

Box 16.3 Fundamentals of a Poster Presentation

- Minimum 24-point text font size
- Headings of a larger font and different color
- Easy-to-read font styles, limited to one or two throughout the poster
- Spaces between sections and paragraphs
- Captions visible and relevant to images, no excessive details
- No overly flashy design
- Colors and contrast that are helpful to those with colorblindness
- Summary and conclusion bullet points, easy to read from 10 feet away

Note: You will not be at your poster the entire time it is displayed. Therefore, make sure the content is clear for all who read it.

16.4 CONCLUSIONS

A poster presentation is a unique format which allows you to present your scholarly work while interacting with attendees in a more personal manner and gaining valuable feedback. Paying close attention to poster design and rehearsing how you will present your research will generate greater interest from viewers, allowing for a more meaningful interaction and a more rewarding presentation experience.

REFERENCES AND RESOURCES

BOOKS
Jacobson K. *Introduction to Health Research Methods.* 3rd ed. Burlington: Jones & Bartlett Learning; 2021.
Lang TA. *How to Write, Publish, and Present in the Health Sciences: A Guide for Clinicians and Laboratory Researchers.* Philadelphia: American College of Physicians; 2010.

ARTICLES
Arslan D, Koca T, Tastekin D, et al. Impact of poster presentations on academic knowledge transfer from the oncologist perspective in Turkey. *Asian Pac J Cancer Prev.* 2014;15(18):7707–7711.

D'Mello A, Flynn O. Respect the poster. *Science*. 2019;366(6466):766.

Dossett LA, Fox EE, del Junco DJ, et al. Don't forget the posters! Quality and content variables associated with accepted abstracts at a national trauma meeting. *J Trauma Acute Care Surg*. 2012;72(5):1429–1434.

Grech V. Presenting scientific work-news media theory in presentations, abstracts, and posters. *Saudi J Anaesth*. 2019;13(Suppl 1):S59–S62.

Goodhand JR, Giles CL, Wahed M, et al. Poster presentations at medical conferences: An effective way of disseminating research? *Clin Med (Lond)*. 2011;11(2):138–141.

Gopal A, Redman M, Cox D, et al. Academic poster design at a national conference: a need for standardised guidance? *Clin Teach*. 2017;14(5):360–364.

Miller JE. Preparing and presenting effective research posters. *Health Serv Res*. 2007;42(1 Pt 1):311–328.

Rowe N, Ilic D. What impact do posters have on academic knowledge transfer? A pilot survey on author attitudes and experiences. *BMC Med Educ*. 2009;9:71

Persky AM. Scientific posters: A plea from a conference attendee. *Am J Pharm Educ*. 2016;80(10):162.

Singh MK. Preparing and presenting effective abstracts and posters in psychiatry. *Acad Psychiatry*. 2014;38(6):709–715.

Wood GJ, Morrison RS. Writing abstracts and developing posters for national meetings. *J Palliat Med*. 2011;14(3):353–359.

CHAPTER 17

Preparing and Giving Effective Oral Presentations

Alice Wang, M.D., Dominik Greda, M.D., Lynne M. Bianchi, Ph.D., and Calhoun D. Cunningham III, M.D.

Tips for Success:

> Create easy-to-read slides that aid audience comprehension.
> Be prepared for audio-visual equipment failure.

Warning:

> You must rehearse many times to ensure your talk fits within the alloted time.

Key Concept: Well-prepared slides benefit both the audience and the speaker.

Presenting your research at an oral presentation session, or a "podium talk," is another common means of disseminating your findings. Much of the advice for creating a successful poster presentation applies to creating a successful oral presentation. Like a poster, an oral presentation tells a story, providing a carefully edited and organized summary of your project.

However, oral presentations also differ from poster presentations in several ways. The most obvious differences are that your study will be displayed on computer-based **slides** instead of a poster board, and you will share your findings only once to a **single audience**. In addition, talks are **timed**, requiring speakers to carefully edit and rehearse to ensure the talk fits into the allotted timeslot.

Most conferences schedule 10 or 15 minutes for each talk with an additional 3–5 minutes for questions. It is important that speakers stay on schedule to match the schedule printed in the conference program as some attendees will arrive to hear selected talks.

A **moderator** typically introduces each speaker in turn. Session moderators also remind speakers when they are running out of time, tell them when their time is up, and help direct questions from the audience. At some conferences, lights on the podium turn green when you begin speaking, flash to yellow when you have 2 minutes left, and turn red when your time is up. **If you have rehearsed your talk multiple times and have the timing down well,** you are likely to find the lights or

DOI: 10.1201/9781003126478-17

moderator's **warning signals more reassuring than stressful**. If you are not well rehearsed, you may find such signals panic inducing.

Note: Some conferences now incorporate rapid-fire sessions with each talk presented in approximately 5 minutes. Others follow the guidelines of PechaKucha, a format in which 20 slides are presented for 20 seconds each.

Tip: An advantage of giving an oral presentation is the potential to reach a broader audience, including many who would not have seen your work in a poster presentation.

Hint: If you indicated to conference organizers that you preferred to present a poster, but your research is accepted for an oral (podium) presentation— congratulations! For many medical conferences, the more impactful studies or topics are assigned as oral presentations to attract a larger audience.

Remember: **Many people find giving a talk challenging**. Public speaking is not a favorite activity for most people, **including the brightest and most competent physicians**. Many of the faculty who instruct residents so well in a small-group setting are uncomfortable speaking in front of an audience. **Know that you are not alone in feeling nervous before a talk**. Suggestions are provided below to help you present without appearing as nervous as you may feel.

17.1 NOTE THE ELEMENTS OF A SUCCESSFUL ORAL PRESENTATION: CLARITY IN SLIDES AND SPEECH

Your talk may be only 10 minutes long, but that is plenty of time to lose an audience. Therefore, you need to pay careful attention to what content you include on your slides and what you say as each is projected. As you plan how to present your study, it is **helpful to think about what makes any presentation engaging and easy to follow** *versus* **one that is distracting and difficult to sit through** (Box 17.1).

Present your slides in a manner that **develops a story** highlighting the study **purpose**, your **findings**, and their **meaning**. As with a poster, you are only presenting what is important for that talk. You will likely leave out some data and secondary findings. You cannot skip data that contradicts what you want to say, but you must be selective in what you show so you build a compelling story that the audience can attend to for the short time you speak. As with designing a poster, you will carefully consider the **organization, font size, colors, layout**, and **spacing of information** on each slide.

It is also important to rehearse your presentation and incorporate strategies that help offset any distracting speaking habits you have. For example, if you are a naturally **monotone speaker**, your slides can offer visual cues to remind you when to highlight information with your voice. If you naturally **talk fast**, you can read a line from each slide to help slow your speech. Similar strategies can be used when presenting a poster.

Tip: **Organized, easy-to-follow slides help offset any speaking errors you make**. Making clear slides that are easy to read will help the audience understand your project and data, even if you end up talking too fast, too quietly, or stumble over your lines. Your slides will also help keep you on script and provide visual cues if you freeze and cannot remember what you wanted to say. Thus, **organized, easy-to-read slides benefit the audience and you**.

Hint: Rehearsing your talk and speaking in a clear, calm, and confident manner is more important than creating "flashy" slides.

Remember: The audience expects oral talks to be brief overviews of data collected from small studies. The audience is not expecting a future Nobel Prize winning discovery, only a **comprehensible presentation spoken in an audible and clear voice**.

Box 17.1 To Improve Your Presentation, Think about What You Dislike

By the time you are a resident, you will have heard hundreds of lectures, numerous presentations from classmates, several seminars, and at least some research talks. You likely can name at least five things you dislike about any presentation. You probably disliked those who read directly from their slides as well as those whose talk did not match the slides shown. You may have been frustrated by those who skipped over slides with comments about, "there is not time to discuss this." Perhaps you recall slides that were impossible to follow because they were too crammed with information, written in small text, or too busy with designs.

You can likely recall speaking habits that made a presentation difficult to follow. Perhaps you dislike listening to speakers who have a monotone voice, those who speak so quietly you cannot make out what they are saying, those who go so fast you cannot process what they are saying, or those who are too nervous to convey a thought clearly.

Before you prepare your talk, write down the things you dislike about other presentations and consider why you dislike them. Then, **avoid doing them to the best of your ability**.

Fortunately, most of things in a talk are under your control. You control what goes on the slides and what you say about each slide. You may talk faster than you should because you are nervous, but with practice that will get better. You may be quiet when you first speak as you gauge the sound from the microphone, but again practice will improve that. Rehearsing over and over (and over) will limit those speaking habits that make it difficult for others to follow what you are saying.

Keep things in perspective: It is okay if your talk is not perfect, just try your best to be clear and comprehensible.

Plan the Order of the Slides: Key Points to Consider

Less Is More

Each slide should include relevant information that can be processed in a minute or two. Content should be clearly visible throughout the room. As with a poster, only the essential information is displayed. Additional information can be included as you speak.

Prepare the Audience

A common outline used when presenting is: **tell the audience what you are going to tell them, tell them, then tell them what you told them**. If done well, this approach reinforces the take-home messages without sounding redundant.

As you present your study, include the same content found in a manuscript or poster, generally following the IMRaD (Introduction, Methods, Results, and Discussion) format. Because this format is so common in medical and science presentations, it helps attendees process content more easily. As you present the content, be sure to highlight and emphasize points that help engage the audience.

> *Tell them what you are going to tell them.* Your first slide will be the **title slide** that includes your name, co-author names, and affiliations. As with a poster, declarative titles are more engaging and informative for the audience and should be used in place of descriptive titles.

You do not read the entire slide to the audience, but say something such as, "Today, I am going to discuss our project about ..." If you are nervous, you can look to the slide and read the title. Often, the first line you speak is the hardest to get out.

Although you will not display your abstract as you do on a poster, it is helpful to begin your talk with an **overview slide** to give the audience a sense of the information you are about to share and the order to come.

- For example, an overview slide could list:
- Background on dementia evaluations
- Development of novel rating scale
- Implementation and findings
- Use in other clinics

As the slide is displayed, you could say, "Today, I am going to discuss our project on dementia diagnoses in adults under the age of 80. After a brief overview of current evaluation practices, I will describe the methods we used to develop a novel detection scale. I will then discuss how we implemented the scale, our results to date, and suggest how this scale can be adapted to other settings."

> *Tell them.* You will then describe your study. Each part of your talk should include a heading to let the audience know where you are in

the talk. Your headings may be Introduction, Methods, Results, and Discussion, or titles that reflect what you are discussing.

For example, when discussing your results, the headings should correspond to the data you are showing such as "New scale detected dementia 8 months earlier than other tools." This helps reinforce the points you want the audience to remember.

Some speakers use icons such as arrows or boxes at the bottom of the slide to highlight where they are in the talk. For example, when discussing the Results, the box or word is bolded or put in a different color:

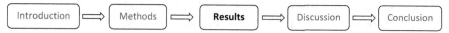

Such **icon guides** should be large enough to see but **should not dominate the slide** or cause the other text to become crowded. If such guides seem more of a distraction than an aid, omit them.

> ***Tell them what you told them.*** Your final slides will be your Discussion and Conclusions. In this final part of your talk, you will briefly remind the audience what you set out to find, what you found, and tie your findings to previous studies where appropriate.

Each slide should clearly state the message you want the audience to remember. If it is important for the audience to know, include it on a slide rather than just stating it in your talk.

INCLUDE THE EXPECTED CONTENT IN EACH SLIDE

An advantage to giving an oral presentation is that you share your findings with a single, larger audience at one time. However, keeping the audience engaged is sometimes more difficult. One way to help audience members follow your talk is to organize slides in a sequence familiar to them.

Introduction: Why Was the Study Done, Why Is It Interesting?

Your Introduction briefly indicates what was done before, what was not known, and what your study addressed. You are not providing a literature review or trying to review details of studies done previously. You only have a short time to present and cannot spend half of it reviewing what was done before. Simply explain enough to set up the rationale for your study.

You will likely have **one or two slides for the Introduction**. If necessary, you may have more, particularly if you need space to keep the text clearly visible. As with a poster, **blank space is *not* a bad attribute**. Blank spaces help viewers find and focus on the text you need them to see.

The last Introduction slide should state the **aims of your study** or **hypothesis**. It should be clear to the audience the purpose of your study and exactly what outcomes you are studying.

Methods: How Was the Study Done?

When you explain your Methods, you need to **provide enough information for audience members to have a clear overview of how the study was done** but you do not need to squeeze in all the details necessary for someone to replicate the study. You should indicate the **study design**, **sample size**, and **statistical analysis**. Include any **novel measurements** or **techniques** you used. For example, if you developed a questionnaire, spend a bit of time describing what is on it. If you used a new antibody in an assay, describe what it binds.

It is often helpful to **present the methods as a list** so the audience can follow the sequence of your work. You can then **expand on each step as you talk**. For example, your slide may state "Incubated in antibody AAb605 (Biopham Labs)," then in your talk you could add, "This is a monoclonal antibody developed in Dr. Bell's lab at the Biopharm Labs that detects the extracellular binding site of protein J. It is the same antibody used in the previous studies I mentioned." Unless characterizing the antibody is a part of your study, you do not need to go into more detail at this point. Audience members who are interested in it can ask questions or contact you after the meeting.

Results: What Were the Main Findings?

This section of your talk includes relevant **images**, **graphs**, and **tables**, and typically includes little or no text other than a heading. **Summarize each finding so an audience member can quickly interpret what is shown on the slide**.

When designing these slides, try to imagine what the images will look like to someone sitting in the back of the room. Also consider whether someone could **read and comprehend the slide during the approximately one minute it is on the screen**. You may have a very nice table that summarizes your data and looks great on your computer screen. Before adding it to your slides, try to digest it all within thirty seconds or one minute. Would you be able to process it if you had not seen it before? Ask someone unfamiliar with your study to look at your images to see if they quickly grasp the content. If they cannot, find a way to simplify any images that were difficult to interpret quickly. You may need to break up information into more than one slide.

Tip: If you include **videos** in your talk, make sure they are compatible on multiple computer platforms and check any conference guidelines for embedding videos. Also, **make sure you can present your talk without the video**. Technical issues sometimes (often) arise so plan for that possibility. Include slides that cover the information from the video, such as still images and summary statements. If the video works, you can review the slides after the video to reinforce your findings or skip over them explaining the slides were included in case the video did not work. The audience will appreciate that you thought ahead.

Discussion: What Do the Findings Mean? What Needs to Be Done Next?

In addition to interpreting your findings for the audience, mention any **next steps** you are planning or **future studies** the field needs to address. You should also briefly indicate **limitations** of your study. To keep your presentation concise, indicate a limitation and state what would need to be done to address that limitation.

Examples:

> Our rating scale may help confirm dementia diagnoses in older adults. Further investigation with a larger sample size is needed.

> AAb605 identified healthy but not precancerous cells in the mouse colon.
> Future studies will evaluate AAb605 binding in other tissues.

Conclusion: What Is the Take-Home Message? What Should Others Remember about Your Study?

End with what you found and how your study filled in a previous gap. Your final slide should be the **main take-home message**, the **one or two points** you want the audience to remember. Keep it simple so those who were distracted at some point can look up and see what they need to remember.

Examples:

> Our rating scale detected dementia in adults over age 80 earlier than existing methods.

> AAb605 identified healthy cells in the mouse colon.

Formally Conclude Your Talk

It is important to formally **conclude your talk**. When you reach your conclusion slide, say something to let the audience know you have completed your talk. The title "Conclusion" provides a visual cue, but you still need to indicate when you are done speaking. Many time speakers just drift off not knowing what to say and then end with "that's it" or some equally abrupt and uninformative statement.

Many presenters use a final slide to help them transition to the end of the talk. Depending on your preferences, conference guidelines, and the conventions of your field, you might put up a slide showing your **references**, a slide of **acknowledgments**, or one asking for **questions**. Whatever final slide you use, end with a statement such as, "That concludes my presentation, thank you for your attention."

Tip: Keep an extra copy of your presentation on a thumb drive and have it ready at the podium. Computer glitches may occur, even at the most highly technological conferences.

17.2 PUT YOUR SLIDES TOGETHER THOUGHTFULLY

There are several software programs that offer slide templates with various background designs, headers, and color options. Some institutions have their own slide templates that incorporate institutional colors and logos. Whatever templates you use, **spend time experimenting with different design options, colors, and fonts, and follow best practices (Box 17.2)**.

DRAFT SLIDE DESIGN AND LAYOUT

Slides should be visually appealing and uncluttered. The text should stand out from any background colors and be spaced appropriately so audience members can read the information from any point in the room. Colors should be appealing and take into consideration audience members who may have **colorblindness**. Make sure key information is presented in a high contrast manner and labeled in a way that does not rely solely on color information. Although computer templates offer an array of styles, there is nothing wrong with simple black text on a white background.

When designing your slides, make each one easy to read and readily comprehendible. Unlike a poster, audience members only see a slide for the time it is projected. They do not have the opportunity to go back to re-read points they missed or want to think about further.

Each slide should be created in a way that allows the information to be processed in about one minute. Also, remember that some audience members will be taking notes and therefore not see the slide the entire time it is shown.

Some software programs provide options for **transitioning between slides**. At times, a dynamic transition is helpful to draw the audience's attention to an important point. However, if used between every slide, the audience is more likely to remember your transitions than your data. As with other aspects of slide design, **use transitions only if attention and comprehension are improved**.

ESTIMATE THE TIME NEEDED FOR EACH SLIDE

To develop a talk that fits the allotted time, it helps to think about how long it will take you to present the information shown on each slide. Some recommend you plan on **two minutes per slide**. Of course, some slides will take longer to describe than others. An introduction with a list of three key points will likely take less time to review than a figure depicting the results from three study groups.

If you have a 10-minute talk and 30 slides, you are going to have great difficulty covering that material effectively in the allotted time. Five slides are likely too few for a 10-minute talk given that some slides will be covered in less than two minutes. Eight to twelve slides may be a good starting point, but the final number will depend on the information you need to present to describe your study effectively.

It is generally best to start with too many slides and then cut back and edit to what is essential.

Tip: Most people are nervous at the time of the actual presentation and thus tend to speak faster than when they are rehearsing. If, during rehearsal, you run through the presentation in 10 minutes, anticipate that you will likely finish sooner than that at the conference.

Hint: Anticipate questions and, where appropriate, include additional slides after your ending slide. This gives you something to display if someone asks a question related to the information on the additional slides.

PROOFREAD
Check each of your final slides carefully for errors. It helps to review them out of sequence and read the sentences on each slide backwards. This will help you identify typographical errors and **evaluate whether the point of each slide is obvious**. Have others check your slides for both errors and ease of comprehension.

Box 17.2   Fundamentals of Slide Preparation

- Minimum of 16-point font; 20- to 24-point font used if possible
- Limited amount of text on each slide—try to use 5–6 words per line with no more than 5–6 lines of text per slide
- Headings of a larger font size and different color to alert viewer to slide content
- Font styles easy to read throughout the room
- Spaces between main points so audience can identify and process easily
- Background colors and text with high contrast and easily read throughout the room
- Colors and contrast helpful to those with colorblindness
- Slides and transitions that are visually appealing, but not too flashy
- Summary and conclusions presented in a manner an audience can process in less than one minute

In the event of an audio-visual equipment malfunction: have your presentation memorized.

17.3 PRESENT YOUR TALK EFFECTIVELY
Audience members are interested in learning new things and are there to hear your presentation. They will listen to many presentations throughout the conference, so it is helpful if you discuss your work in a simple but engaging manner. You do not need to make jokes or entertain the audience, but you should think about how and when to add comments that complement and reinforce the information on your slides.

REHEARSE

You will need to practice your talk multiple times to optimize both your wording and timing. You will **practice to yourself** and **in front of others**. When you present to others, if possible, practice in a large room to get used to what it will feel like at the conference. You should practice by yourself before and after presenting to others. It feels awkward to talk to yourself, but it really helps (**Box 17.3**).

Each time you rehearse, schedule enough time to run through your talk more than once so you can start over and revise as needed. Conference talks are generally short so it will be easy to find the time to practice at least once a day in the weeks leading up to the conference.

Note: Do not wait until a day or two before the conference to begin rehearsing.

Tip: Identify and practice strategies that help you speak clearly. Put cues on your slides to remind you when to slow down, add inflection to your voice, or pause for emphasis. **Revise your slides after rehearsing, if necessary**.

Hint: Practice not turning your back to the audience to read off a slide. Your slides should only be used as a visual aid to enhance the key points of your oral presentation.

FAMILIARIZE YOURSELF WITH THE ROOM AND PODIUM

Once at the conference, go to the room where you will present. If possible, go the day before your session and try out the audio-visual equipment. The day of the conference, arrive early for your session, introduce yourself to the moderator and audiovisual assistant, and confirm that your talk is ready to go.

ANTICIPATE QUESTIONS

You can likely anticipate questions people might ask about your study. **Be sure to practice answering the questions out loud**. Having an answer in your head and stating it clearly and concisely are two very different things. Rehearsing answers will help you stay calmer and appear more confident at the conference. Have colleagues and mentors suggest additional questions and encourage them to ask questions during your rehearsals so you can get used to "thinking on your feet."

At the conference, listen carefully to each question asked so you do not inadvertently answer something you anticipated being asked rather than the actual question. It is **helpful to repeat the question** asked by a member of the audience. This allows you to clarify what is being asked and helps those in the audience who did not hear the question when it was asked.

If a question arises that you do not know the answer to, indicate you do not know. **Do not attempt to create an answer if you do not have one**.

Tip: Try not to say, "That is a good question" to every question. It starts to sound rehearsed and insincere after a while.

Remember: The audience should have a clear sense of why your study is interesting. It is okay if your study is not interesting to every person in the room. The people in the audience are there because they are interested in the topic of the session and therefore will likely have some interest in what you are going to present. Your job is to share your enthusiasm to help hold their attention for the 10–15 minutes of your talk. If your data are not relevant to some audience members, they should understand why they are relevant to you, your institution, or your community. Some of your data will be very specific to the patient populations you see and may not be as pertinent to larger or smaller institutions or communities. **Every audience member should grasp the study rationale, agree the data were collected correctly, and concur that the findings are relevant to the population studied**.

Dress for Success

Dress appropriately and professionally. Although the type of conference dictates the dress code, whatever the standards, when speaking at a podium, look professional. Most presenters at medical conferences wear business-style clothing such as a coat and tie or skirt, dress, or slacks with a jacket. Follow the norms of your conference and subfield, but never appear too casual.

If you purchase new clothing specifically for your talk, wear it once or twice before the meeting so you are more comfortable. The day of the talk is not a good time to discover an itchy seam.

Tip: Some conferences are held in warm and sunny places that convey a vacation-like atmosphere. Avoid the temptation to wear shorts, sandals, or swimwear even if you see others dressing that way.

Hint: You want others to remember your data, not your clothing, or lack thereof.

Note: The same advice on dressing for success is given for presenting a poster.

Box 17.3   A Presenter's Perspective: Dealing with a Fear of Public Speaking

Most people who are afraid of public speaking think their fear is worse than that of others. "Yes, others get nervous, but not the way *I* do." At least one of the authors of this chapter felt that way throughout post-graduate work. Despite efforts of teachers and mentors along the way, who encouraged and reassured and offered helpful tips, the author was convinced it was impossible to overcome such extreme nervousness and avoided every assignment that required speaking in front of a class and declined opportunities to present at meetings. One day sitting in a seminar, looking forward to a talk by someone working in a similar field, it finally dawned on the author that being nervous was a huge distraction to the audience. The only thing that was remembered about that talk was the nervousness of the speaker and how everyone felt a mixture of sympathy for the speaker and frustration that the point of the talk was lost. **Recognizing that the audience is interested in your slides and data can help you focus more on the mechanics of the talk and less on your reaction to giving the talk.**

Once you decide you do not want to be remembered for your shaking hands and trembling voice, but for your data, you can **focus on what you need to do to compensate for your innate nervousness.**

The author rehearsed over and over until the talk was memorized down to the hand gestures and places to pause. By the time the real talk came, only the first slide was presented with a shaking voice. The talk was still delivered faster than it should have been, and the laser pointer was rather shaky at times, but the talk was understandable, and the data were the focus of the presentation, not the speaker.

You can create your slides in such a way so there is a key line or phrase that helps you remember what you want to say. You can highlight key points in ways that help slow a fast pace or signal where to add some inflection to an otherwise shaky, monotone voice. You can also think of a line on each slide as a comfort phrase, a **cue to help calm you down and pause if needed.** You can read directly from the slide or use slightly modified wording. Only you will see them as comfort cues, the audience will just see text. Each slide you get through is a step closer to the end so you can breathe a little better each time you complete an identified phrase. **Drawing attention to details of a slide also helps keep the audience focused on the slides and not you.**

Most large **rooms will be dimly lit** so the slides are visible. Knowing you cannot be seen clearly can also provide comfort.

Remember: The audience is there to see the slides, not you. If you do not do anything terribly distracting or dress in anything unusual, the audience will be focused on your slides.

17.4 CONCLUSIONS

Practice makes perfect. Your first few oral presentations will feel the most nerve wracking and take the most time to perfect. With more experience, however, talks become easier and may eventually feel like second nature to you. Listen to as many other presentations as possible and learn from others—many national and international conferences will highlight or showcase work from prominent leaders in your field. Some will give talks worth emulating. Note the formats and styles that help an audience process information easily.

There were many tips and notes shared in this chapter. The most important tip to remember, however, is this: enjoy it! Be proud of your accomplishments and enjoy sharing your work with others. One day, it will be your turn to share your first experience and guide others on how to prepare for their conferences.

REFERENCES AND RESOURCES

BOOKS
Jacobson K. *Introduction to Health Research Methods*. 3rd ed. Burlington: Jones & Bartlett Learning; 2021.
Lang TA. *How to Write, Publish, and Present in the Health Sciences: A Guide for Clinicians and Laboratory Researchers*. Philadelphia: American College of Physicians; 2010.

ARTICLES
Alexandrov AV, Hennerici MG. How to prepare and deliver a scientific presentation. Teaching course presentation at the 21st European Stroke Conference, Lisboa, May 2012.
Blome C, Sondermann H, Augustin M. Accepted standards on how to give a medical research presentation: A systematic review of expert opinion papers. *GMS J Med Educ*. 2017;34(1):Doc11.
Grech V. Presenting scientific work-news media theory in presentations, abstracts, and posters. *Saudi J Anaesth*. 2019;13(Suppl 1):S59–S62.
Monzó Gardiner JI, Secin FP, González Enguita C. Fifty ways to improve presentations in urology. Cincuenta consejos para mejorar las presentaciones en urología. *Actas Urol Esp (Engl Ed)*. 2020;44(1):14–18.
Waljee JF, Larson BP, Chang KW, et al. Developing the art of scientific presentation. *J Hand Surg Am*. 2012;37(12):2580–2588.e82.

CHAPTER 18

Organizing a Successful Local or Regional Conference

Diann C. Cooper, Ph.D., Jeffrey Esper, D.O., and Lynne M. Bianchi, Ph.D.

Tips for Success:

> Work with a reliable planning team.
> Establish clear submission and presentation criteria.
> Keep good notes and meet all deadlines.

Warning:

> Failure to consult with the appropriate institutional officials regarding procedures, contracts, or continuing education requirements can cause unnecessary setbacks and complications.

Key Concept: Create a conference with a clearly defined purpose that meets the needs of the target audience.

Medical conferences are a great way for clinicians and researchers to interact, share data, and discuss ideas. Conferences range from single afternoon sessions featuring poster presentations to week-long conferences with keynote speakers, oral presentations, and poster sessions. Some conferences highlight recent research discoveries, some emphasize advances in patient care, and many offer continuing education credits. Whatever the size and structure, every conference requires a group of individuals to plan the programming and organize the daily events.

As a faculty member, you may initiate or help organize a local or regional conference or serve on a planning committee for a national or international conference. Residents may assist a faculty member, or serve on a planning committee for a local, regional, or resident-focused conference.

This chapter outlines common practices for faculty and residents charged with putting together a small- to mid-sized local or regional conference. Topics addressed include selecting a conference **planning group**, preparing a **timeline**, and defining the **purpose**, **target audience**, **location**, **conference format**, and **budget**. Advice for **advertising**, attracting **presenters**, **selecting** speakers, and **avoiding common mistakes** is also offered.

Note: Organizing a conference is a form of faculty scholarly activity.

DOI: 10.1201/9781003126478-18

Tip: There are many ways to assist with organizing a conference and, as with other forms of scholarly activity, it is beneficial to focus on areas that are of interest to you, fit your ways of thinking, and do not exceed your available time.

18.1 WORK WITH A RELIABLE CONFERENCE PLANNING COMMITTEE

Organizing a conference requires time and attention to detail. One of the best ways to ensure a successful conference is to work with others committed to creating a positive experience for attendees. Whether a formal committee or a small group of volunteers, the planning group must be dedicated to organizing a professional, worthwhile event.

To accomplish all the necessary goals, a diverse skill set is required. Every planning group should include members with interests or expertise related to the conference content, event planning, and marketing. If you are tasked with organizing such a group, **identify colleagues with expertise you lack**. It is helpful to include at least one person who has successfully planned other events. Include individuals knowledgeable about the academic content and colleagues in administrative offices at your institution. Choosing colleagues with innate organizational skills is also wise. Individuals from marketing, communications, library, and medical education departments also have skills and experience beneficial to a planning group. If you are unsure who to invite, **talk with others to get suggestions**. Also think about your network of contacts; is there someone who has attended numerous conferences that might offer helpful suggestions?

COMMON PLANNING COMMITTEE MEMBERS

Content Experts

Individuals familiar with the topics covered at the conference. These members may have general medical and research knowledge or be experts in a specific subfield. Examples include faculty and senior residents from your department, members of other residency programs at your institution, a research director, and university faculty.

Administrative Experts

People knowledgeable about the institution's protocols and procedures. Every planning group needs someone to submit requests for room reservations, audiovisual equipment, printed materials, and off-campus services. Your department's administrative assistant and program coordinator may be good choices to assist with such efforts, if permitted by their job descriptions.

Members of the Target Audience

Those who would benefit from the event. Who do you envision coming to the conference? Students? Residents? Physicians? Nurses and other health care professionals? Including members of the target audience on the planning committee helps ensure the needs and interests of the broader group are addressed.

Marketing and Communication Personnel

People to help promote the event. Whether a large or small conference, you need to inform others about it. For small institutional conferences, flyers and emails may be all that are required. A colleague with some artistic talent might create and disseminate such documents. For larger conferences, external marketing targeted to individuals, institutions, or professional societies may be needed. You might want additional advertising *via* social media, websites, radio, or television. When broader marketing is required, identify someone in your institution or community with contacts and experience in these areas.

Tip: Consider the diversity of the target audience. Include committee members who can review marketing approaches to ensure no one is unintentionally discouraged from attending. Invite members to address issues of accessibility for attendees with hearing, mobility, vision, or other difficulties.

Hint: If organizing your first, local conference, keep your planning group small and include people you know are organized and efficient. Try to find people who can fill multiple roles, such as a content expert with mobility challenges who has helped organize other conferences.

Note: Some conferences require a conference planner, an individual or company with event planning expertise. Professional societies, for example, often contract with companies to organize national conferences.

Remember: If you need conference planning assistance, the continuing education, medical education, or similar office or department at your institution may have personnel or materials to guide you.

18.2 MAKE THE MOST OF YOUR PLANNING MEETINGS

Your group will meet several times prior to the conference. The first meetings are used to identify needs, set goals, and assign tasks. Subsequent meetings are used to review progress and check that everything is addressed in a timely and proper manner. An example planning scenario is provided in **Box 18.1**.

Depending on the size and location of the event, you may start planning more than a year before the conference date. Although there is no defined number or required length of planning meetings, it is essential to keep **accurate records of all discussions, correspondence, and assignments**. Among the first considerations for any conference planning committee are to:

Define the Conference Purpose

Why are you organizing the conference? Is it to share research results or discuss current clinical practices? Is it to provide opportunities for students or trainees to present? Do you want to bring in experts from outside your region to share new information?

The committee should **articulate why the conference is needed**. Are residents required to present at a conference prior to graduation? Have faculty expressed interest in learning more about their colleagues' research? Are there recent advances in a clinical area that should be shared?

Identify Who Should Attend

As you define the purpose and significance of your conference, think about the **speakers and target audience** you want to attract. Who would be motivated to come, given the conference goals? Who would benefit from the event? Will the committee invite speakers, accept submissions from those interested in presenting, or both? Are members of the planning committee expected to present?

As you discuss potential speakers and the target audience, you simultaneously **consider the event location, dates, and budget**, as these impact who ultimately attends the conference.

For example, the planning group may determine all health care professionals in the country would benefit from the event, but your resources and budget accommodate only a few hundred attendees. Thus, you would revise your target audience to a subset of health care workers, such as those from specific institutions or professional societies.

If the purpose of the conference is to have senior residents present their final research projects, the planning group would schedule the conference before June graduation ceremonies.

Choose an Effective Format for the Program

How should information be shared, given the purpose, location, budget, and timeframe? Poster presentations and podium talks are common formats. Virtual presentations, moderated panel discussions, and discussion groups are also frequently used. Nearly any format can be implemented provided it suits the audience and attracts participants.

Discuss Which Format(s) Would Best Meet the Needs of the Target Audience

Poster presentations are a great way for presenters and attendees to interact. The format encourages discussions and fosters networking. Several posters can be set up at the same time, allowing more presentations at a given session. When done well, attendees can process content from several posters in a single session, allowing them to learn a lot in a short period of time.

Unfortunately, not all posters are done well. If attendees find that many posters are difficult to follow or feel presenters did not communicate effectively, the conference may be viewed as unprofessional. Listing requirements for poster size, format, and content often improves the consistency and quality of posters.

Podium presentations or lectures reach a larger audience at once, but limit networking opportunities. Presentations range from about 10 minutes to an hour in length. Some are intended to provide an overview of one's latest research; others are intended to educate the audience on a topic of interest.

Many conferences include a **keynote speaker** who covers material related to the theme of the conference. Well-known speakers often attract audience members from outside your institution and region. An honorarium and travel expenses are usually offered to keynote speakers; therefore, the planning group will need to consider these expenses as they work through the final format of the program.

Virtual presentations with speakers and attendees connecting through an online platform are becoming more common. Because the time and expense required to travel to an in-person conference prohibits many people from attending, virtual platforms increase access. If the entire conference is held virtually, conference organizers save money on expenses such as venue fees and food costs.

While accessibility and costs savings make virtual presentations attractive, many speakers and attendees find it challenging to stay engaged and note that opportunities for networking are limited.

Some conferences offer hybrid models in which some speakers and attendees gather in person, with others joining virtually. Organizers must take care to ensure a positive experience for both on-site and remote participants.

Moderated panel discussions often include a group of experts sharing opinions on a stated topic or answering questions from the moderator and audience. Some panels include slide presentations by panel members. Depending on the conference goals, the moderator's primary role may be to monitor speaking times or to act as liaison between the panel members and the audience.

Discussion groups or workshops allow attendees to share thoughts on a particular topic. The audience breaks into small groups to complete an assignment that is then shared with the larger audience. This format often works well when the goal is to brainstorm and share new ideas, such as those regarding educational initiatives. Attendees benefit most when the sessions are organized around specific tasks and a moderator provides structure and summarizes discussion points.

In weighing the various options, the planning group will **develop a programming structure that meets the goals of the conference**. A full-day conference with a keynote speaker, followed by concurrent podium and poster sessions, might be desirable for some. For others, time and budget constraints might support a half-day conference of poster presentations. Others may find morning podium talks followed by afternoon discussion groups best. The important thing is for the committee to **identify which formats are most helpful to the target audience, given the planned content and available resources**.

BUILD A PROGRAM THAT FITS YOUR BUDGET

Budgetary constraints are a reality every planning group must face. Having a provisional budget before the first meeting is helpful. There is no point in planning a fantastic conference that can never come to fruition.

If the planning group determines the program would benefit from something that exceeds the existing budget, **identify potential funding sources to offset costs**. For example, the committee may decide to charge registration fees to generate income or ask vendors who exhibit products at the conference to purchase food. There may be grants from your institution or professional society available, or another hospital or university may be willing to co-sponsor the event.

Note: Be certain to check with the appropriate offices at your institution before accepting any financial support from an exhibitor or other commercial entity. There may be institutional regulations or continuing medical education protocols that restrict the size and nature of donations that can be accepted.

Tip: Do not underestimate the importance of consulting with institutional officials prior to accepting donations to support your conference.

The Venue

Where do you plan to have your conference? Does this site charge a fee? If so, does the fee include use of audiovisual equipment, poster board stands, registration tables, chairs, and other items necessary for the conference? If not, are those items available for an additional fee? Do you need to hire others to provide those items or pay those who set them up for the conference?

Wherever your hold your conference, you will likely have some costs associated with using the space and materials. Your institution may not charge you to use a large room for an afternoon of poster presentations, but you will likely need to pay personnel to configure the room prior to the presentations and remove items when the conference ends.

Audio-Visual Needs

For many conferences, this is one of the largest expenses incurred. Audiovisual support may be included in the venue fee. Alternatively, you might need to pay for equipment rental and hire technical support personnel.

Refreshments

The length and format of your conference often dictates what sort of food and beverages to provide. Should you provide coffee, tea, soft drinks, and water for the audience? Will you need to offer a snack break or meal? Does the venue offer catering? Will they require you to use their catering, or can you hire off-site caterers? Does the caterer charge per person or plate, or a flat fee? Are there options for those with dietary restrictions or preferences (vegetarian, vegan, gluten free, sugar free, Kosher)? What are the charges for those options?

Providing food or beverages can use quite a bit of one's budget. The planning committee must balance what would be most appreciated and least wasteful. No one wants to run out of beverages or snacks during the first hour but there is no benefit to purchasing items that are later discarded. Where possible, develop a mechanism for attendees to indicate dietary restrictions or preferences prior to the event so the correct amount is available.

Tip: Consult with caterers or colleagues who have hosted similar events to get a sense of how much to supply.

Keynote Speaker

Keynote speaker fees range from hundreds to thousands of dollars. You will need to confirm the speaker's fee and estimate travel, lodging, and *per diem* expenses. Some speakers may be willing to waive their honorarium if travel expenses and conference registration are covered.

In some cases, bringing in a well-known speaker attracts more attendees. If you charge a conference registration fee, speaker-related costs may be offset by the increased attendance.

Note: Your institution may have rules regarding the amount of any honoraria offered and the types of expenses covered. **Always review institution protocols and reimbursement procedures before offering honoraria and travel expenses.**

Tip: A keynote speaker does not need to be an internationally recognized expert. You simply need a knowledgeable and engaging speaker that the audience will appreciate hearing.

Hint: Not all well-known experts are engaging speakers. Get feedback from others before inviting anyone to give the keynote address.

Moderators

Will you ask others to host or moderate any sessions? Will these be local volunteers, or will you invite outside speakers to assist? Will you offer an honorarium or reimburse travel expenses for any moderators? Does your institution have financial guidelines for paying or reimbursing moderators?

Advertising Costs

How do you plan to inform your target audience about the conference? For a small conference, email notifications may be sufficient. However, for others, direct mailing may be needed. If that is the case, what materials will you mail? Who will prepare and print them?

Mailing Lists

If you are sending printed information to the homes or offices of potential audience members, you can identify the appropriate postal zip codes and make a request to purchase mailing lists from a professional organization. Some lists are state- or profession-specific so you would include the costs of the desired mailing lists in your budget.

Printed Materials

Small conferences held at your institution will likely require, at a minimum, printed flyers and program handouts. You must therefore budget for printing or photocopying those materials. Some regional conferences need professionally printed announcements and program booklets. Your institution may have on-site printing or contract with a specific vendor. If not, the marketing or communications department at your institution may have a list of contacts.

Hint: Creating and producing program materials can cost a great deal and take several months to complete, so consider available options and costs early in the process.

Presentation Awards

Some conferences, particularly those highlighting student and trainee work, offer awards for the best presentations. Monetary prizes, gift cards, trophies, or certificates may be awarded. To budget accordingly, the committee should determine early in the process what, if any, awards will be given.

Tip: An administrative or educational department at your institution may be willing to sponsor the awards.

Hint: Confirm that award evaluation criteria are consistent with submission and presentation requirements. Identify judges who will provide helpful, impartial evaluations.

ESTABLISH A REALISTIC TIMELINE AND COMMUNICATE OFTEN

The easiest way to develop a timeline is to decide when you want to have the conference, then work backward. In general, the larger the program, the more time you will need. For example, at least a year of planning is required for a conference that involves invited speakers, regional advertising, and an off-site venue. In contrast, smaller, on-site programs are often arranged in a few months.

It is helpful to **meet on a regular basis and increase the frequency of meetings closer to the program date**. For example, if you are planning on-site poster presentations at the end of April, meet once a month in January and February, then weekly in March and April.

A key to a successful program is frequent and clear communication. Planning meetings do not have to be grueling, time-consuming events. What is important is that committee members talk with each other often, attend to all tasks, and confirm all institutional procedures are followed (see also **Box 18.2**). Many meetings will be short or involve only a subset of the committee. Some discussions can be held *via* video conferencing or email. For every meeting, **designate someone to keep track of assignments, due dates, and the committee member(s) responsible for each activity**.

Tip: If you find yourself working with a shorter-than-ideal timeframe for an off-site conference, develop a smaller program. Leave the audience with a good first impression, then expand the program the following year, if desired.

18.3 FOLLOW ALL PROTOCOLS WHEN AWARDING CONTINUING EDUCATION CREDIT

Health care professionals must earn continuing education (CE) credits to maintain licensure. Physicians, both allopathic and osteopathic, earn continuing medical education (CME) credits. Other health professionals may earn CME or other continuing education units (CEUs). The number and type of credits necessary are determined by discipline and the state or country of practice.

Organizing a conference that awards CE credits can increase attendance and revenue. If your conference content is appropriate, it is often worthwhile to consider offering CE credits. However, there are numerous **regulations that must**

be followed, so someone on the committee must be responsible for ensuring all standards are met.

Your institution, or a co-sponsoring institution, must be approved to offer CE credits by an accreditation body, such as the Accreditation Council for Continuing Medical Education (ACCME), American Osteopathic Association, or American Nurses Credentialing Center (ANCC). Fortunately, many hospitals have a designated office available to assist program organizers and check that CE credits are calculated and awarded correctly. This office can also verify that the required language is placed in program advertisements and announcements, that attendance is monitored and documented accurately, and that necessary files are maintained for continued accreditation.

Tip: If your institution does not have a CME or CE office, check with other nearby hospitals or medical schools to learn more about the procedures and requirements for offering CME or CEU. Another institution may be interested in co-sponsoring your conference if it is of interest to their staff.

18.4 DETERMINE ELIGIBILITY, SUBMISSION, AND PRESENTATION REQUIREMENTS

Guidelines are necessary, whether planning a small conference or a large event. Standards and requirements are articulated so committee members, presenters, and attendees know what to expect. **Without standards, a conference will appear disorganized and unprofessional**.

Before announcing the conference, the committee will establish requirements and presentation guidelines so those interested in presenting can prepare appropriately. Work with the planning committee to **establish clear eligibility requirements, submission procedures, and presentation expectations**. In developing submission and presentation criteria, consider practicalities such as space, time, and financial constraints. For example, if there is space for 50 posters, should you accept 100 posters and organize morning and afternoon presentations, schedule two sessions over a 2-day period, or select only 50? If you accept only 50, how will posters be selected? Also, consider the conference goals and content needs. If the purpose of the conference is to give residents presentation experience, the committee may decide not to accept presentations from medical students or faculty physicians. Alternatively, all submissions might be accepted, with a session devoted to resident presentations.

Hint: The benefits of clearly defined submission and presentation criteria far exceed the time it takes to define them.

ELIGIBILITY

The committee must establish what topics and formats are suitable for the conference and who can present. Listing inclusion and exclusion criteria is helpful in keeping the program focused and consistent with the conference goals.

What Can Be Presented?

The committee considers which topics and forms of scholarly activity fit the purpose of the conference and lists relevant information in the conference announcements to guide those interested in presenting.

The planning committee might discuss whether clinical and basic science studies are eligible, whether case reports or quality improvement projects should be included, or whether studies with preliminary data can be presented.

Who Can Present?

What credentials are required for presenters? Is the conference limited to work by physicians or are all health care professionals and scientists eligible to present?

Depending on the nature of the conference you may only allow students or trainees to present. Conversely, you may prefer that no students or trainees present or allow students and trainees to present posters, but reserve podium talks for senior faculty.

Note: If the conference is sponsored by a professional society or provides continuing education credits, check whether all or a portion of the presenters and planning committee must be members of that professional society or have a certain degree (M.D., D.O., Ph.D.).

How Will Eligibility Be Confirmed?

Once you determine eligibility criteria for content and presenters, decide how you will confirm that eligibility is met. You might design a checklist that includes topics, format, and presenter qualifications. You may require a *curriculum vitae* to confirm degree status.

Note: If organizing a conference that awards continuing education or other credits, work with the continuing education office to establish how speaker eligibility is to be confirmed and documented.

Tip: Some biographical information should be collected from all speakers, such as name, degree, and current institution affiliation. This information is usually included in the program book. For keynote speakers, you might include information on educational background, publications, and areas of expertise. This information can also be used when introducing the speaker.

Hint: Including contact information in the program book helps attendees develop a network of contacts.

Submission Review Procedures

How will the committee evaluate submissions? Will you require abstracts or applications to be submitted? Who will review these submissions? The entire committee or a subcommittee? Do you need more than one subcommittee to review submissions on different topics?

What are the *specific* review criteria? When organizing a conference, "I like this one" is not an evaluation. You need clear, consistent criteria that all reviewers agree upon and can justify if questioned.

A checklist with eligibility criteria and a scoring rubric is helpful. Reviewers can check if specific items are present and score some content on a Likert scale. If abstracts are reviewed, include the same criteria you posted for presenters, such as word count, font style, font size, and formatting structure (e.g., Introduction, Methods, Results, Discussion, and Conclusion).

Note: Include a space on the checklist to list abstract topics. This becomes helpful for assigning presentations to a suitable session.

Tip: If you can only select a subset of the submissions, identify the ineligible and poor-quality submissions first, then rank the remaining submissions.

Hint: Ineligible and poor-quality abstracts are usually the easiest to identify.

Presentation Expectations

Directions and guidelines are necessary for a successful conference. Presenters must know how to organize their talks and prepare and submit their materials. For example, those preparing posters must know the size and orientation of poster display boards so they can print a poster of the correct size. They must be given formatting requirements for headings and text size so they can organize the content properly. Those giving oral presentations need to know how long to speak, what audiovisual equipment will be available, and what computer software or operating systems are compatible. If materials are to be submitted prior to the conference, instructions for doing so need to be given. **The committee works out these details prior to announcing the conference.**

If the conference includes poster and oral presentations, the committee must also decide whether presenters will select the format they prefer, or if the committee will assign a format. If the committee chooses the format, criteria for assigning each submission must be developed so both reviewers and presenters are aware of the procedures.

18.5 REVIEW POST-CONFERENCE EVALUATIONS

Feedback helps guide future planning groups. To learn what worked and what did not, many conference organizers ask attendees to complete an evaluation form that includes a mix of multiple choice, ranking, and open-ended questions. Many evaluation forms include sections for attendees to rate aspects of the conferences on a Likert scale and space for additional comments related to those ratings.

Conference evaluations may **request feedback** on the overall **content** relative to the purpose of the event, the appropriateness of **speakers** for the audience, the conference organization and **programming**, the **food** service, quality of **exhibitors**, and the location and comfort of the **venue**. Many evaluation forms include space for suggestions on **what should change** for the next conference.

A member or subcommittee of the planning group summarizes the evaluations for the rest of the group. It is helpful to meet within a week of the conference to review feedback and make notes for the next planning committee as such information contributes to the needs assessment for subsequent conferences.

Note: Evaluation forms for conferences offering continuing medical education (CME) or other professional credits usually require specific questions or formats. Consult with your continuing education office to ensure all necessary information is included.

Tip: There are many examples of program evaluation forms online and in the literature. Modify existing forms to suit your needs.

Box 18.1   An Organizer's Perspective: Frequent Communication and Good Notes Are Essential

It helps to know what to expect when planning a conference. Volunteering to assist on a planning committee is a great way to learn the many steps and challenges involved. The sample scenario below provides an idea of what to expect when organizing a small conference at your institution.

Imagine you and a group of colleagues are organizing a conference for graduating residents and advanced practitioners (APs) to present the results of their senior projects. Dr. Dowell-Vasquez a member of one of the residency departments, is elected as chairperson of the planning committee. Two other physician-faculty members (Drs. Ayoub and Wienckowski), a nurse practitioner (Ms. Jiang), a senior resident (Dr. Xavier), the residency program coordinator (Ms. Muller), the department administrative assistant (Mr. Kaiser), and a member of the hospital marketing team (Ms. Sills) are included in the planning committee. The agenda of the first meeting is:

Agenda: First Planning Meeting
  Introduction of planning group
  Introduction of idea
  Purpose
  Needs assessment
  Audience
  Format
  Presenters
  Date, Time, Location
  Food
  Advertising
  Cost
  Timeline

The administrative assist, Mr. Kaiser, records minutes of the meeting as follows:

Minutes: Planning Group Meeting October 7	**Discussion Leaders/Responsible Party for Follow-up**
Agenda Items	
Introduction of idea, introduction to group members	Dr. Dowell-Vasquez
Purpose—to provide resident and APs with experience presenting and discussing research	Dr. Dowell-Vasquez
Needs Assessment—past graduates noted they have little experience presenting research results and feel underprepared to present at national conferences	Dr. Dowell-Vasquez
Target Audience—medical and nursing staff, residents, students rotating at hospital	All
Committee agrees, no one is excluded but content to be geared to the target audience	
Format—committee voted to hold poster presentations to allow for the maximum number of speakers	Dr. Ayoub will send presenter eligibility information, poster submission guidelines, and poster formatting requirements to all graduating residents.
	Program coordinator, Ms. Muller, will identify hospital contact(s) to forward information to other eligible presenters.
Presenters—all graduating residents and APs must present; other hospital staff and trainees are eligible to present	Subcommittee of faculty will review and select abstracts for presentation by January 26.
	Biographical information needed for each presenter. Dr. Xavier will create form; Mr. Kaiser will email to presenters.

Date, Time, Location—hospital conference room, April 30. Session 1: 12:00–3:00 pm; Session 2: 5:00–8:00 pm.	Ms. Muller to reserve room. Mr. Kaiser to schedule appropriate personnel for room set-up and clean-up.
Refreshments—Water available in conference room; Coffee, tea, cookies, and fruit outside of room one hour before sessions begin, removed after second hour	Ms. Muller and Dr. Wienckowski will contact other departments to solicit contributions to cover refreshment costs. Mr. Kaiser will work with Ms. Jiang on food selections and ordering; will determine if hospital catering or outside vendor to be used; get estimate of costs.
Advertising	Ms. Sills and the marketing department will create flyer to post and design an email announcement with graphics to send to hospital employees. Dr. Ayoub will develop a list of email contacts to invite faculty and students from local university.
Cost	After an estimate of food and beverage costs is obtained, all residency and AP departments will be asked to contribute (Ms. Muller, Dr. Wienckowski). Dr. Dowell-Vasquez will ask research director to cover cost of printing posters, and medical education office to cover set-up and clean-up costs.
Timeline—Committee discussed dates for future meetings and follow-up	Next meeting October 14 at 10:00 am

Proposed Timeline: Approved October 14:

Date	Action	Committee members
October 7	**1st planning meeting**	Dr. Dowell-Vasquez
October 14	**2nd planning meeting**—review eligibility criteria, poster formatting guidelines, biographical information forms; finalize timeline	All
November 10	**3rd planning meeting**—updates on room reservation, room set-up/clean-up plans, refreshment costs; finalize advertisements; discuss conference evaluation form	All

November 30	**Approved advertisement sent** out to hospital and university personnel	Dr. Dowell-Vasquez emails committee with updates
January 15	**Abstracts due**, submitted to Dr. Dowell-Vasquez	Mr. Kaiser creates single document and sends to faculty subcommittee for review
January 18–25	**Abstracts reviewed** by faculty subcommittee	Faculty review subcommittee
January 26	**Abstract selection meeting**: Final abstracts selected	Faculty review subcommittee
January 29	**5th planning meeting**—assign presentation times for each accepted submission; review status of food and beverage plans; department contributions	All
February 3	**Presenters informed** of acceptance and given presentation time. Those not accepted informed of committee decision, encouraged to submit to future conference.	Dr. Dowell-Vasquez composes emails indicating whether submission was accepted or declined. Program coordinator sends appropriate email to submitting authors.
March 1	**Biographical information forms due**	Mr. Kaiser collects, Dr. Xavier reviews; Mr. Kaiser sends reminders or revision requests as needed
March 15	**Posters submitted** for review prior to printing	Faculty review subcommittee
April 5	**Final posters sent for printing**	Program coordinator collects and sends to printer
April 7	**Food ordered**	Mr. Kaiser
April 14	**Program booklet photocopied**	Marketing provides cover, Ms. Sills copies.
April 21	**Updates** from all areas	All via email communication
April 29	**Review room arrangement**	Drs. Dowell-Vasquez and Xavier
April 30	**CONFERENCE DAY** Set out program books and evaluation forms before sessions begin	Drs. Dowell-Vasquez, Xavier and Wienckowski
May 7	**Final meeting**—review program strengths and weaknesses; prepare needs assessment for next committee	All

> **Box 18.2   Faculty Perspective: Important Considerations**
> **That Are Often Overlooked**
>
> When speaking with experienced conference organizers, many note lessons they learned the hard way. Some mistakes led to poor presentations, some wreaked havoc on the budget, and others led to legal disputes. To make your conference run smoothly, include at least one experienced conference or event organizer on your planning committee and keep this advice in mind:
>
> **Avoid choosing speakers based on friendship or politics.** Choose speakers with a reputation for giving a good talk.
>
> **Tell presenters what operating systems and software programs are compatible with available audiovisual equipment.** Technical difficulties and conference delays arise when materials cannot be used with available equipment.
>
> **Inform presenters that any videos or animations must be embedded in the presentation.** Do not rely on internet connections to access videos or animations as service is often unpredictable.
>
> **Have a back-up keynote speaker** in the event someone is delayed or must cancel at the last minute.
>
> **Pay attention to the dates of other conferences** so you do not schedule a conference that conflicts with other obligations of your target audience.
>
> **If reserving a block of hotel rooms for out-of-town attendees, reserve half the expected number.** Make sure your conference will not be held financially responsible for unreserved rooms.
>
> **Be cautious about offering to provide copies of slides or other presented content to attendees.** Presentations may include copyrighted material that cannot to be distributed without permission.
>
> *Always* **have the appropriate office at your institution review contracts before you sign.**
>
> *Always* **have the appropriate office at your institution review drafts of program materials before they are printed and distributed.**
>
> *Always* **have the appropriate contact person at your institution review procedures for sharing presentation materials.**

18.5 CONCLUSIONS

Conferences are vital to the career of every researcher and health care professional. Conferences bring together people with similar interests, stimulate new ideas, support networking and collaborative opportunities, and often provide continuing education credits. Quality conferences are needed and appreciated by others.

Organizing a conference is a challenging but rewarding experience. To create a quality conference and minimize complications, work with a reliable team that includes experienced conference planners and institutional administrators.

If your group has a clear purpose for the conference, meets regularly, communicates frequently, keeps good notes, stays on budget, and develops clear guidelines for presenters, your conference is likely to be a success.

REFERENCES AND RESOURCES

BOOKS

Billings DH and Halstead JA. *Teaching in Nursing: A Guide for Faculty.* 5th ed. St. Louis: Elsevier; 2016.

O'Shea K. *Staff Development Nursing Secrets: Questions and Answers Reveal the Secrets to Successful Staff Development.* Philadelphia: Hanley & Belfus, Inc. Medical Publishers, 2002.

ARTICLES

Buring SM, Bhushan A, Broeseker A, et al. Interprofessional education: Definitions, student competencies, and guidelines for implementation. *Am J Pharm Educ.* 2009;73(4):Article 59, 1-6.

Schmitt M, Blue A, Aschenbrener CA, Viggiano TR. Core competencies for interprofessional collaborative practice: Reforming health care by transforming health professionals' education. *Acad Med.* 2011;86(11):1351.

RESOURCES

Become Accredited ACCME
- https://accme.org/become-accredited

How to Transfer CME Credits for AMA
- https://edhub.ama-assn.org/pages/applications

Institute of Medicine (US) Committee on Planning a Continuing Health Professional Education Institute. *Redesigning Continuing Education in the Health Professions.* National Academies Press, 2010.
- https://www.ncbi.nlm.nih.gov/books/NBK219811

Interprofessional Education Collaborative
- https://www.ipecollaborative.org/

Resources for CME Sponsors from American Osteopathic Association
- https://osteopathic.org/cme/cme-sponsor-accreditation/

World Health Organization. *Framework for Action on Interprofessional Education and Collaborative Practice.* WHO Press, 2010.
- http://apps.who.int/iris/bitstream/handle/10665/70185/WHO_HRH_HPN_10.3_eng.pdf;jsessionid=17C5B24D8E7E83B99B3E0441A3199007?sequence=1

Index

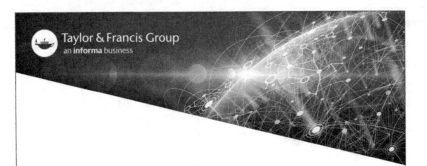

Printed in the United States
by Baker & Taylor Publisher Services